I0424720

Welcome

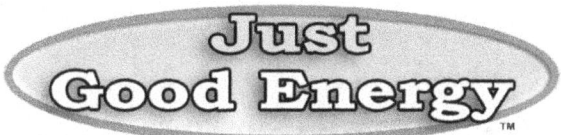

Transition to an All Natural, High Energy Lifestyle

by Rebekah Winquest

The information contained in this book is provided solely for general educational purposes and should not be construed as medical advice for the treatment of specific illness. Each person and situation is unique. No book can replace the diagnostic expertise and medical advice of a trusted physician. Please be certain to consult with your doctor before making any decisions that affect your health, particularly if you suffer from any medical condition or have any symptom that may require treatment.

Transition to an All Natural, High Energy Lifestyle

Library of Congress Catalog Number: U1-281-871
ISBN: 1453700889
EAN-13: 9781453700884

Copyright © 2006 by Just Good Energy, Rebekah Winquest
Printed in the United States of America

All rights reserved. No part of this book may be copied or reproduced for commercial purposes without the written permission of the publisher.

Copy edited by Shawn Winquest

Published by
Just Good Energy
Malibu, CA

www.justgoodenergy.com
Email: info@justgoodenergy.com

ACKNOWLEDGEMENTS

Appreciation to:

Shawn, my husband, who encouraged me to believe I have something to say.

Lou and Judy, my mother and father

All of the health pioneers who have dedicated their lives to research, educating and creating for the benefit of many.

JUST GOOD ENERGY

www.JustGoodEnergy.com

JGE exists as a reflection of Rebekah Winquest's mission to educate, empower, and guide you on your path to optimal health, helping you achieve maximum, natural, and sustained physical and mental energy that your body is truly craving so that you are experiencing every day to the fullest. You can also visit Bek's blog at JustGoodEnergy.com to get her weekly recipes, videos, product analysis, and her up-to-date information on nutrition and natural living.

Rebekah Winquest
Holistic Nutritionist, Herbalogist, Chef and Recipe Designer of Natural Foods & Meals
She continues to consult, publish, and research while counseling clients and managing her nutrition and natural foods company, Just Good Energy.

DEDICATION

I would like to dedicate this book to my husband, our families, and my spiritual father, John Robert Stevens.

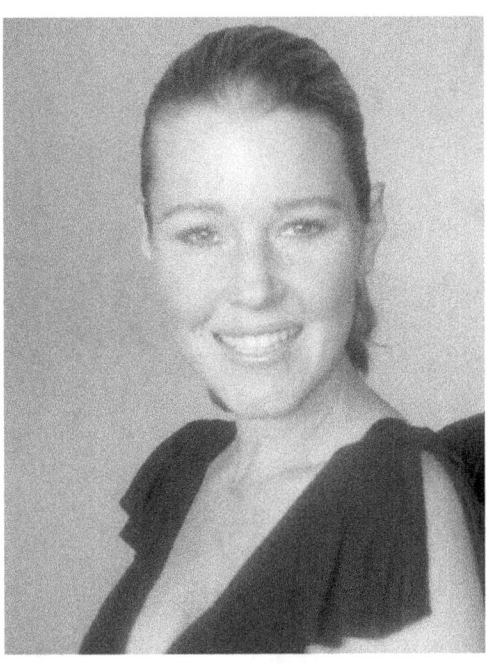

There is not a singular timetable or solution for all to make their personal change, but there are philosophical guard rails, practical guide posts, and fundamental disciplines that combine to help you in what is essentially a continuous journey—that which leads to your own optimal lifestyle and health.

My personal journey to a total lifestyle change began at an early age. I had always been a curious child—especially for the elemental world. I developed a fascination for both the practical and profound influences that foods have on our health. I began my education by reading every book on nutrition I could find, digesting the many points of view by those who have dedicated their lives to the field. I continued my education at the Clayton College of Natural Health where I received my Bachelors of Science in Holistic Nutrition. I then set out to transfer that theoretical knowledge to practice to help family, friends and clients get healthy, and most enjoyably in the kitchen where I can express my creative energy. I see daily how this knowledge improves the health of my family and clients. Most encouraging is how the changes in our diet improve and expand our positive energy.

I truly believe that each and every one of us can develop an earthly balance through foods and smart, truly natural supplements to reach a level of energy that enables us to experience and enjoy every day to the fullest. I want to share my knowledge with you. The approach of this book is to simplify what can appear as a daunting task. I pray that is what I've achieved on your behalf. Best wishes and good luck on your journey.

~ Rebekah Winquest

Table of Contents

Part III – Setting Up Your Kitchen - 141

Part IV – Soaking & Sprouting - 155

INTRODUCTION

Today, there are all types and varying degrees of mass diets, step-by-step eating strategies, and weight loss programs that are marketed to be all-inclusive health and wellness solutions for many. Unfortunately, a total one-stop-shop solution for optimal health does not exist. We are all unique individuals and must be treated as such. Our uniqueness is what makes us human. Each of us is a masterpiece in our own right because there is not one other person in the whole world just like us. This is a fascinating and profoundly beautiful thing, but this also means that we are each responsible for becoming the gatekeeper to our own health. To own and commit to our health means that we must seek out and set in place fundamental, but flexible tenets that guide our lifestyle and diet through a journey of education, empowerment and personal discovery.

Most of the programs marketed as silver bullet solutions are designed for people to lose weight. Almost all of them have little to do with improving the participant's overall health, and everything to do with capitalizing on a person's obsession with losing the pounds. Achieving one's optimal weight is critical for multiple reasons, but true good health can only be gained through a balance in lifestyle. Losing weight is a tactical result of an overall transformation strategy. If you craft a lifestyle that is balanced, your optimal weight should be reached naturally. How do you know if you are out of balance? The answer to that complex question can typically be found by first asking a simple question, 'How do I feel?'

A lifestyle is a unique compilation of personal choices, both a subjective and shared total sensory experience. What, when, where, and how we eat combine to have a critical influence on our lifestyle. I admire and follow most all practices of Raw Foodists, Vegetarians and Vegans. The fundamental difference in my approach is that it is completely open to individual discovery and without limitations on choice. I do not believe in limits because a limit prevents me from exploring, which might prevent me from discovering the right choices for me. An open approach such as this means that we focus on the personal choices that influence a lifestyle that will ultimately suit our own personal balance, which might include elements of many dietary practices. The resulting lifestyle is fueled by the combined effort of those choices, which will define our physical and mental energy. The quality and level of that personal energy is, in my view, the most critical indicator for *how we feel*.

If what we put in our bodies has the most influence on our energy then certainly we must do everything we can to understand foods, and how they affect us holistically. Focus on developing a passion to learn as much as possible about foods, their functionality, energy value, and how everything we eat and drink affects our body, mind, and emotions. That way, you can make a transition to a lifestyle that will give your being the most sustained and positive energy.

In this book, I've simplified complex nutritional principals into a language that anyone can understand. We are first going to establish the foundation or "launching pad" to help you make the choices and decisions for making the change in your diet. I will explain how to optimize your body for proper digestion through understanding enzymes and how they relate to raw versus cooked foods. I will teach you how to cleanse your body of past and daily toxins. I lay out in detail the simple steps to get you started on your gradual transition to a more live and plant-based diet through understanding the categories of foods and the strategic phases of transition. I then give you the guidelines on what to eat depending on the time of day so that you have optimal good energy throughout your day-span. You will learn about the importance of exercising your body, mind, and spirit during your transition. You will learn how to prepare your kitchen for a good energy lifestyle. You will become a healthy shopping expert by learning exactly which foods to shop for, and will gain specific and critical information you need to sort through the countless supplements available at your local health food grocer so that you do not waste time and money on products that may be harming you more than helping you. The guide has much more, and exists holistically as a comprehensive road map to take along on your life path.

This guide will excite and motivate you to move forward on the path to positive energy and overall health. The guide will be with you as you explore and discover the potential of your body, mind and spirit, and how foods can be such a fun and integral part of your lifestyle and well-being.

To Your Health!

Rebekah Winquest

PART I
MAKING THE CHANGE

Chapter 1
The Foundation

Chapter 2
Let's Talk About Enzymes

Chapter 3
Cleansing

Chapter 4
Making the Transition

Chapter 5
Exercise: The Best Friend of Nutrition

Chapter 6
Exercising the Spirit

Chapter 7
Planning Ahead for your Energy Demand

CHAPTER ONE

The Foundation

Regardless of your age or state of health, you can make a healthy lifestyle change now that will improve your quality of life. It is indeed possible for change to happen by accident, but that isn't the kind of change we are referring to. We are talking about change that is dependent on purposeful motion. That motion, regardless of the type, requires energy. Therefore, energy, that is, positive energy, is the key to making a balanced lifestyle change. Good energy is the means to that end, and is also the end goal in itself.

What does *energy* mean? The word *energy* comes from the Greek *energeia*, or activity. The wise Greek philosopher, Aristotle, was one of the first to define this term writing that, "Every existing thing has an *energeia* that maintains it in being and is related to its end of function, or *telos*." He defined a body's potential or capacity for action as its *dynamis*. He observed and was one of the first to refer to energy as the body being "at work" en route to – or at – that *telos*, or a specific function.

The known world is comprised and made up of energy. We, as a moving part of the one universe are all about energy—not the obvious sources we are all acquainted with—solar, wind, oil, gas, coal, but an underlying energy at the base level of creation that causes all matter to have form and substance. Energy, in essence, is that which is born out of the vibration of the molecular structures that comprise everything.

As humans we are also comprised of energy. We are, in effect, energetic beings. And because of this, our atmosphere and peers affect us more than we have ever understood. Whether it is the food we eat, the water we drink, the air we breathe, the music that fills us with joy and guides our emotions, the clothes we wear, the colors we are drawn toward, or our personal viewpoint and paradigm of what we call "reality", everything is energy, and that energy has a dynamic affect upon us. In this 21st century, we are only now beginning to understand and accept just how much we are energetic beings, and how our interaction with nature, the world about us, the environment, can have such a dynamic affect, both on us and upon this planet on which we subsist.

As I've begun to explain, energy is not only found in the created form we see about us, but energy is created in the thoughts we think, and in our personal viewpoint of what is real, what is possible, and what is not. Who defined what is possible?

Our minds are magnets for limitations created by our knowledge and experiences; definitions based on our five senses of perception, but perception is a subjective experience. After all, our perception revolves around our faith in the spirit and our personal view of our self that is the center of *our* world. Much if not of all of our limitations have been picked up somewhere along the way; influenced by a combined connection with our family, faith, peers, education, sciences, and our relative experiences on this sojourn. All of this "information" is constantly being beamed at us, causing us to make decisions, every moment of every day. It is so much easier to say, "I can't do this", than to confront our belief system, and say, "Why not?" I can do this. What sets apart the "doers" from those on the sidelines?—a belief system that does not accept limitation. Your reality does not have to be limited. To be sure, these limitations or barriers can and should be overcome through natural means, which is the only way to avoid artificial or synthetic realities that only create a muddled awareness.

Our balance and energy is more thoroughly viewed through a holistic lens. The holistic approach is to first recognize and appreciate our body as a working "whole", and not just a series of individual parts. To subscribe to a holistic approach means breaking the bond of the two-dimensional view that a singular action produces a singular reaction. An action almost always results in a set of reactions that causes varying consequences. Each action, reaction, and consequence must be thought of uniformly in order to find a true and sustained solution.

Delineating our own energy dichotomously as "good" or "bad" is relative to what one's own perception is of oneself. Each of us is an individual with our own unique soul, DNA signature, experiences, and collection of ideas of what their future might behold. Therefore, each of us is ultimately responsible for choosing and defining how we are going to shape our journey that will involve many interdependent paths.

We each have a unique balance necessary to completing this journey. To find one's balance along the way, one must traverse through a process of exploration, discovery, empowerment, and often a total lifestyle change depending on the degree of imbalance that can develop along the way. Balance and energy are bound together in a constant expression, a dance we might call it, and as we know there are many forms of dance. Our ability as humans to be consciously aware allows us to examine the choices we make in our lives on the degree of positive energy created for ourselves and spread to others. We can also investigate how our own energy balance affects the natural elements that we come in contact with that are as alive and as active as we are. In other words, our relationship with the earth and all that lives upon it is as important as the connections we make with our fellow humans.

All food has an associated energy. In many religions and cultures, it is commonplace to bless, meditate, or pray over the food before eating. You have the ability to create within your food a synergy and harmony that will be both a blessing and strength to your body, soul and spirit—even more so if the food you eat is not "dead" but has a life giving energy to it that can be thought of as a vibration. When you think of energy, you might think of the positive aspects, but much of the food consumed in America today is what I would call a negative energy food. Rather than give life, it takes away life. Rather than help lift your personal vibration, it works to bring your vibration and energy level down. Rather than cultivating a higher awareness of the world about us, and who we are inside, the negative energy of the fast and dead foods that are so prevalent today work to cloud and diminish our inner clarity and awareness. So, in totality, rather than add to your vibration, negative energy foods can actually diminish your life-force.

All foods in their "raw" state have life. Generally the more "dense" the food substance is, the slower that food vibrates and the lesser the energy it actually has. Some foods, what we call today "super-foods", such as pomegranate, acai, wheat grass, algae, and goji berry have incredibly high amounts of energy and vibration, and actually work in harmony with your system to bring a higher level of vibration to you.

A person's vibration is the amount of electrical energy that the body puts out and needs throughout the day. I first came across this exciting relationship years ago when reading Tony Robbins excellent book, *Living Health (pg. 34 cc 99 ARC)*. Mr. Robbins explains the profound idea that every single entity in the world vibrates at its own unique frequency? He goes on to explain how science has documented that every plant, food, animal, person, organ, cell, thought, color, etc., has its own vibration, which can be measured in megahertz (MHz). The body's main organs (heart, brain, lungs, etc.) should vibrate at about 70 MHz, when it is healthy. Chocolate cake only provides 1-3 MHz of energy. Most of the fried burgers at fast food outlets give a whopping -5 to 3 MHz – pretty sad for a "complete meal". Those happy meals aren't so happy! There are "high-vibration" foods, which can add high amounts of energy to our own. For example, raw almonds have 40-50 MHz; green vegetables and wheat grass have 70-90 MHz. For you hopeless romantics, the scent that roses give off actually has a vibration of 300-350 MHz (that's why girls love them so much). So it appears that natural, plant-based foods give off an incredible amount of energy, where processed (sugary, starchy and fried) and fast foods give little to no energy. There are many common fast foods and candies that actually give off a negative amount of energy!

So we vibrate at one level and foods vibrate at different levels—what is the connection? If you need 70 MHz of energy on a daily basis and you live off of junk food, and soda, you are creating an energy-deficit crisis in your body. When you are sick, stressed, or exhausted, and your body is already low in energy, how can you expect it to work overtime and heal itself? The body can't without breaking down. That is how we get illnesses, gain weight, become lethargic, loose muscle mass, and lower our IQ. Your body will age faster if you do not give it the good energy it needs.

I want to challenge you to begin to analyze your diet and energy within the holistic context of your total lifestyle as opposed to only using the traditional measurements of calorie intake and BMI as the primary metrics for success. Those metrics are key measures as you move forward with your change, but they are not the only metrics. Moreover, our obsession with the metric of the calorie can make us vulnerable to certain elements of the food and beverage industry that often strive to manipulate our perception to control the choices we make. A basic example of this misinformation is that a food that is low in calories doesn't necessarily mean it is nutritious. I think most folks understand that, but it is easy to get confused when examining labels in the market. We will expand on this subject and much more in the chapters to come. For now, please just understand that you are the gatekeeper, and are responsible for asking all the questions to those who profess authority on your behalf. That includes the FDA, profit driven weight loss programs, and any entity deployed by the government or corporations to determine what is right for your health. You cannot afford to outsource that duty, and why would you want to? What I will show you is that to own the role as gatekeeper is the most empowering position you will ever hold.

Transforming to a natural lifestyle is not just about making your life longer because lifespan is an ambiguous term. Quality of life is what we are talking about, and we measure quality on how you feel each and every moment. Why limit yourself to thirty healthy years when you could have eighty or even a hundred? Why have any limits? Empower yourself with the energy to make every living day the best it could ever be because you are perceiving and experiencing with the highest level of sustained life-force so that each day builds on the other as you continue on your journey, while enjoying each moment on your path. This is your life and regardless of what hand you've been dealt or dealt yourself early on, it is a continuous course of learning, adjusting and optimizing. Your health is a trinity of body, mind, and spirit. When all three are working optimally, you can reach a holistic balance that allows you to live on the highest levels of vibration.

Each food and beverage that you put into your body, whether directly or indirectly serves a function that will cause the organs and systems to respond. You can think of each and every food you eat as more than just a substance to ingest to satisfy your hunger or emotional desire, but rather to explore the nutrition and overall energy value of foods, and then to discover how food can be used to provide maximum energy for the physical and mental activities of everyday living, and how foods have and can provide preventive and healing properties. The functionality of a food is dependent on how it was grown or produced, how far it is from its natural state, whether it is a single food such as an apple or a combination of ingredients, the time of day it is eaten, and is ultimately a sum of the individual values of each ingredient added to it, and how each of those 'whole' foods enhance health and the quality of life.

So how do we make the most conscious choices throughout our day? In an ideal lifestyle, every meal would be a meditative, contemplative time, shared with other people, but life has become so fast paced that for most, that ideal has become impossible, especially while at work and zipping through the daily schedule where the deadline trumps the diet. The solution to staying balanced within a fast pace lifestyle is planning ahead. Planning ahead for your energy demand will empower you as the gatekeeper, and will help you break free of any dependence on compromised foods or restaurants for your daily energy and overall nutrition.

What I am asking you to do as you move forward is to open up your mind to how the way you eat is a lifestyle and not just a diet. I am not asking you to change who you truly are, but am inviting you to realize how much of a positive influence food can be on your overall being. Opening the mind is the first step to making a change. Once your mind is open, you can allow in the building blocks necessary to develop a solid foundation for what may be the most exciting and important change you ever make.

Is your mind open? Good. Let's begin.

CHAPTER
TWO

Let's Talk About Enzymes

The Role of Enzymes

To understand any lifestyle of eating and what makes your body tick, you need to understand the concept of enzymes.

What are they and what do they do for you?

What jump-starts your day? What is that generator inside your body that keeps you going and provides energy? Enzymes, which occur naturally in all living things, are the catalyst for every cell to do its job. Every single function that takes place within our body, including pumping our blood and the growth of new cells, requires enzymes to begin, carry out, and complete the process. Enzymes maintain our health and proper body function. There are three categories of enzymes, which activate every single biochemical process: Digestive, Metabolic and Food.

Digestive enzymes, mainly produced by the pancreas, are the active agents responsible for the digestion of food. Digestive enzymes properly break down the food we consume, allowing the nutrients to be absorbed and distributed throughout our blood stream. Without these enzymes, food would putrefy and rot in our intestines, producing excessive toxins and fat storage. Also the body would not be able to absorb the nutrients that were originally available in the food, thus creating mal-nourishment.

Metabolic enzymes have earned the title, "Foundation of life". Every chemical reaction that takes place in the body is dependent on that specific metabolic enzyme. Every single cell that makes up tissue, muscle and organs is reliant on that specific enzyme reaction to give it life and energy. Our body's ability to function, heal and repair when injured, fight diseases, and grow is dependent on that specific enzyme to catalyze or jump-start the process. Think of enzymes like a key to a car. Without that key, the car won't start and perform.

Food enzymes are naturally available in the raw foods that we consume. They are a gift from nature, aiding the digestion and absorption process. Foods high in enzymes—raw, soaked, and sprouted foods—not only pre-digest themselves, allowing you to get the most nutrients from the food, but those highest in enzymes -- sprouted and fermented foods and plants -- add to the pool of enzymes in your body, helping you to live longer and healthier. Only foods that are raw, or not heated above 115 degrees—the temperature at which enzymes die—contain enzymes that help maintain or add to our enzyme supplies.

All three of these enzyme categories make up essential building blocks that regulate the state of our health. When either of these enzyme categories is depleted, the body becomes more susceptible to illness, and when they are gone completely, our life has expired.

The bodies' capacity for enzymes, which may be designated as the "enzyme potential", is obviously fixed and limited. To assume otherwise would deny natural law. Since the day of birth, our body begins producing digestive and metabolic enzymes and as we age we produce less and less. It has been proven that by the age of forty, we are only producing half the amount of enzymes that we need to sustain a healthy and vital life.

Let us paint a picture of the "enzyme potential": If the body is constantly producing enzymes for digestion, it has no time to produce the metabolic enzymes needed to heal, rejuvenate, energize and detoxify. This unhealthy state in the body gradually creates a lethargic, depressed, disease-prone system that is doomed to pre-mature termination. The body is truly made to regenerate and continually heal itself. However, without the chance of having metabolic enzymes at its disposal, one cannot expect the impossible. It takes more energy to digest food than almost any other process in the body so we must always take a conscience stance when eating and measure ahead so that we are aware of the amount of energy the body is going to have to expend in order to properly digest what we feed it. Simply put, the reason people walk around tired after eating a large meal is that all energy is being dedicated towards digestion.

Most of the food consumed by the American public is refined, processed, overcooked and dead. When you eat cooked or processed food you are draining your enzyme pool. Rather than giving you life, this "lifeless food" takes your life, bite by bite. Over a lifetime, you become less and less productive, less energetic and much less healthy.

Anthony J. Cichoke writes in his influential text, Enzymes for Enzyme Therapy,

"If the world was created by divine power, one realizes that life on it was created through enzymes, the elemental energy source or basic life force."

The Solution
Now that the need for digestive enzymes has been established, let us explore the various ways to incorporate them into our diet. The body is constantly in the state of digestion. Therefore, enzymes are continuously exhausted. To preserve our potential we need to reduce internal digestive enzyme production. One of the easiest ways to do this is to limit the number of digestive enzymes that our body needs to break these meals down. By making less digestive enzymes we will ultimately make more metabolic enzymes daily.

There are three ways to preserve this potential. All three are based on reducing the amount of energy that we spend on digestion. The optimum choice is to eat more raw foods as discussed previously. The second choice is to eat moderately and more frequently throughout the day, and never over-eat. Basically, if we consume less in one meal, the body has to work less, producing fewer enzymes. The third choice is taking a high quality digestive enzyme supplement with every meal. Of all "supplements" available in the market, digestive enzymes are one of the most essential and life-giving products one could take. An enzyme blend should specifically include:

- ❖ Protein enzymes (protease, bromelain, papain)
- ❖ Carbohydrate enzymes (amylase, alpha-galactosidase, maltase)
- ❖ Fat enzymes (lipase); fiber enzymes (cellulase)
- ❖ Dairy enzymes (lactase**)**

We are very fortunate to have these products available to us. Taking enzymes could be the difference between a shorter and unhealthy life and one that functions optimally and energetically. Digestive enzymes should be taken with both cooked (enzyme-less) and raw (enzyme-rich) foods. The reason being that not only do enzymes help to break food down, but they also help to absorb the nutrients from the food. Your entire nutrition strategy can fall short if there is a problem with mal-absorption or any nutrient deficiencies.

Supplemental protein (protease) enzymes can also be used to help heal conditions such as inflammation, Candida, immune deficiency, tissue damage, and toxicity. Protein enzymes should be taken on an empty stomach if they are being used for a specific health issue that does not include digestion. Bacteria, fungus, viruses, and parasites invade our blood stream under the protection of a protein covering. Since the invaders of our blood system are protein, it would make sense that ingesting protease (protein enzyme) on an empty stomach would help break down that protein coating. The immune system can then take action on eliminating the bacteria or unwanted foreign invader, thus purifying the blood.

Finally, enzyme deficiency is also a leading factor in obesity. This may sound odd, but a person can be overweight and malnourished at the same time. When a diet consists mainly of dead, processed and enzyme-robbing foods, the result is inflammation and fat storage. It takes at least thirty minutes for ingested food to receive enzymes and begin the digestion process. In the mean time, food ferments, rots, creates acid, and is stored as fat cells. As a result, most of the nutrients that were present in the food have been lost. Enzyme potential is also essential to a body's metabolism. If a system is deficient in enzymes, the metabolism is unable to function properly. One of the crucial functions of metabolism is burning fats. If fats aren't burnt, they are stored as visceral fat cells, most likely creating that beloved abdominal spare tire.

I began researching enzyme companies about six years ago and came across the company, ENZYMEDICA. Enzymedica produces high potency vegan enzymes that are at least six times stronger and more effective than any other company I have researched and tested.

Understanding Raw Foods

Why are Raw Foods Important?
Only live, fresh, and unrefined foods regenerate the body and prevent the depletion of its own life-giving supply of enzymes. A diet comprised primarily of cooked and processed foods will create sluggish, congested cells incapable of vibrant living. Diets high in animal protein and saturated oils interfere with the natural wisdom cells need and possess to direct the optimum functioning of our bodies' regenerative abilities. Whereas a fresh, uncooked, plant-based diet allows for optimal cellular regeneration as nature intended.

Simply put, cooked food (over 115 degrees), refined and processed foods, dairy, an excess of red meat, and chemicals (alcohol, caffeine, tobacco, preservatives, and pesticides) takes away from the natural energy of the body, which equates to energy loss. Raw and vibrant foods including uncooked fruits, vegetables, sea vegetables, raw nuts and seeds, dehydrated/raw grains and legumes are all enzyme-rich, and add to your body's pool of energy, which equates to energy gain.

Finally, the human body is about 70% water, so it makes perfect sense that our body desires at least half the amount (ideally 70%) of its daily food intake from raw foods, which are generally high in water content.

Raw Foods....
- ❖ Increase energy, vitality, and an overall sense of well being
- ❖ Cleanse the body of accumulated toxins and waste
- ❖ Contain the highest concentration of vitamins, minerals, and nutrients
- ❖ Help prevent disease through proper cellular regeneration

Learn more about specific raw foods and how to apply them to your daily diet in Chapter 9.

Choose Organic

Your produce, grains, legumes, seeds and nuts are only as nutritious as the ground they come from, so whenever you can, buy organic. In order for a food to be labeled "organic" the soil it came from must be free of chemicals and pesticides for 10 years, and the growers must only use organic fertilizer. The organic matter used by organic growers brings fertility back to the soil, which has been neglected by conventional farmers. While the rise of pesticides and synthetic fertilizers has increased tenfold in the last forty years, crop losses due to insects have doubled. Organic methods, on the other hand, build up the soil, creating stronger, more disease-resistant plants.

Most people would be surprised to know that while 10% of the pesticides ingested in our country come from produce, 90% are found in animal products. Produce is treated with pesticides a set number of times during its growth, while factory farm animals are fed pesticide-laden crops regularly. The pesticides eaten daily by the animals are absorbed into their tissues and stored there. When you eat these animals or the milk products they produce, you are consuming concentrated doses in uncontrolled combinations of many of the most deadly chemicals ever known.

Eating organic is the only way to avoid toxic chemicals, and guarantee that you are receiving the nutrition that nature intended. You will find that organic produce is much more flavorful. If you are home growing, buy organic seeds, fertilizer or composts. If you choose to eat processed foods, buy organic, and if you choose to eat meat, buy free range.

The Importance of Soaking & Sprouting

The History of Sprouting
The use of soaked and sprouted foods has been dated back as early as 3000 B.C. According to early records written by the Emperor of China, sprouted beans were prescribed for complaints such as edema, muscular cramps, digestive disorders, weakness of the lungs, and skin and hair problems.

More recently, Purdue University recorded that sprouted foods were an excellent high-quality protein source. Dr. Tsai of Purdue considers them to be one of the most perfect foods known to man. Sprouted wheat was found to be, by itself, one of the only known foods that could sustain the life and health of experimental animals. Soaked and sprouted nuts, seeds, legumes and grains are at their most nutritious state, full of live enzymes, and easily digested and absorbed.

Soaking

There are several good reasons to soak your grains, nuts, seeds or legumes. One is that the higher the water content in a food, the better it is for us. After a food is soaked approximately 6-12 hours, the inhibitors that prevent it from digesting well are washed away and it is able to release the enzymes, proteins and carbohydrates that are vital to our survival. Soaking nuts and seeds also reduce the fat content about 40-50 percent, increasing the protein and mineral content, and are therefore preferred over just raw nuts and seeds. When a food is changed from a dried, dormant state by soaking, it becomes a live, easier to digest plant.

Sprouting

Now that we have soaked the food, why sprout? Soaking brings the plant to life; sprouting completes the cycle. Sprouting creates an enzymatic transformation; the plant actually goes through a chemical metamorphosis. The plant becomes a concentrated form of nutrients, which becomes the most "alive" source of food available. Sprouting causes the plant to develop its full enzyme capacity that enables the plant to pre-digest itself.

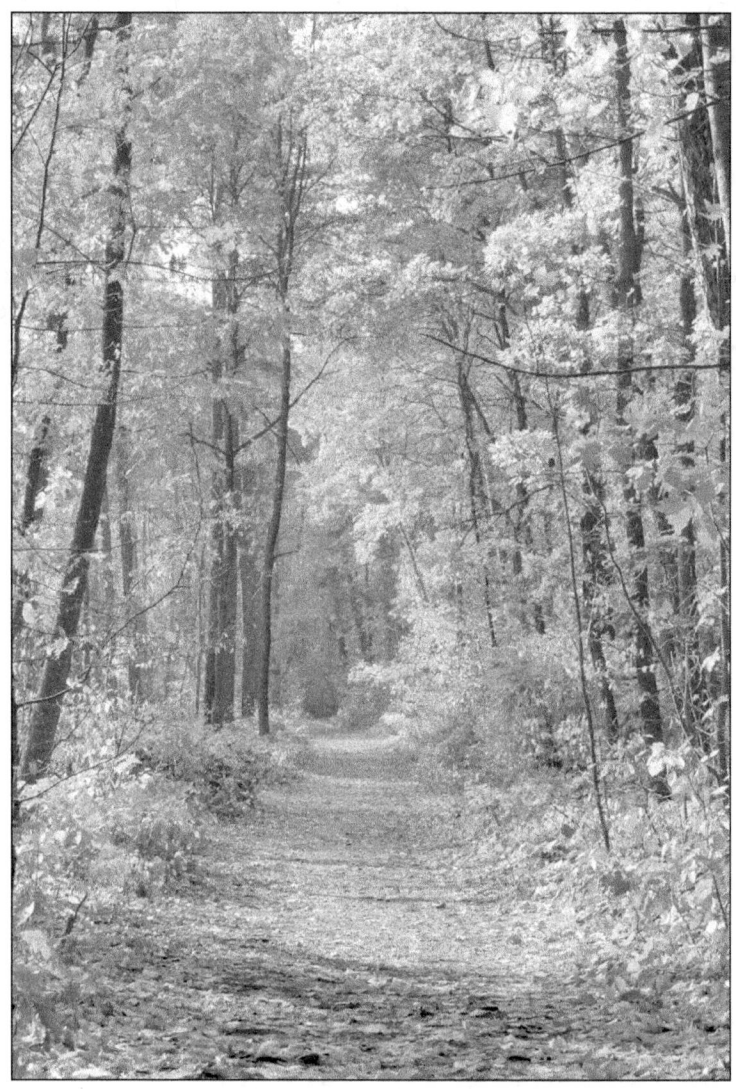

"I am convinced digestion is the great secret of life."
~ Sydney Smith

CHAPTER THREE

CLEANSING AND WATER

Your body receives the nourishment your food contains through the absorption of the nutrients as the food travels through the intestines. To properly assimilate these nutrients, the intestinal pathway must be clear. Water cannot flow freely through clogged pipes! When the lining of the intestine is blocked by improperly digested food, we receive only minimal benefit.

The fasting process is best used and thought of as a vital tool, giving the body the opportunity to transform itself physically. Fasting aids your ability to change your habits and lifestyle during the detoxification process. Resting from foods and allowing the body to process what it has already stored, is the ideal sequence to correct the imbalance caused by our congestive and excessive eating behaviors. Congestion within the body is a result of eating excessive "bad" fats, animal and processed foods. Refined, processed or chemically treated food cannot be properly digested. This "so-called" food will stagnate in the intestine, causing a release of toxins that lingers in the digestive system and enters the bloodstream. Any foreign substance that your body does not recognize as a nutrient is classified as a toxin. Therefore, pasteurized foods or those processed by adding chemical preservatives, nitrates or hormones cause a multitude of problems.

Any food, except raw food or super-foods, will wait in the upper stomach for a half-hour to an hour while the pancreas sends digestive enzymes to break it down. This waiting period is a prime time for the toxins in the food to begin infecting the body's vital systems and bloodstream. Over time, our bodies suffer a toxic buildup and are in great need of a thorough cleansing.

As surprising as it may seem, overweight people suffer from malnutrition because their intestinal tract is clogged. When our diet includes a variety of raw foods, especially green grasses and sea vegetables, then we are receiving the proper amount of roughage to help us clean out and at the same time supply our body with the enzymes to help fight toxic buildup and disease.

There are many types of cleansing programs, but to simplify, I will break them down into two categories:

I. Herbal Supplement Cleanses

❖ Involve taking herbal supplements with some food intake

II. Juice fasting / Raw food / Super-food Cleanses

❖ Involve drinking juices and/or a combination of super-foods and raw foods
❖ Incorporate alkaline water during your cleanse and up to 2 weeks max for cleansing purposes.

I prefer the cleanse that requires juice fasting and super/raw food intake because this option is in my view, gentler on the body, mind, and spirit. I believe a cleanse should be as natural and comfortable experience as possible. The discomfort will be unique to one's present state of health. Basically, the more you have to cleanse, the more challenging it is for your body to cooperate. Below are two levels of cleanse, a three-day and eleven-day.

A three-day cleanse is ideal for the first-time, or as part of your yearly health maintenance. It will help you to reduce weight, relax stiff joints, relieve constipation, and of course assist in the elimination of toxins. The length of a cleanse depends on your individual health needs, and the unique requirements of your lifestyle. It can be difficult to implement a cleanse longer than three days if you have a demanding schedule.

I recommend three days minimum to make an impact on your body, but you can certainly stretch your cleanse further. You can customize your cleanse for as many days as you would like. There is no hard rule. The length depends on how much toxic build up you have to cleanse, and how long your schedule and health requirements allow you to go. Always check with your physician before your cleanse if you have unique health issues.

Please set a goal of cleansing your body a minimum of two to three times per year. These cleanses do not have to be long—a three-day juice fast is sufficient. These fasts will help keep you clean, are beneficial for illnesses, and help rid you of unwanted fats or toxins.

On the following pages are the steps to a three day and longer eleven day cleanse.

The Three-Day Cleanse

❖ First thing in the morning on each of the three consecutive days, drink 8 to 16 ounces of prune juice or lemon juice and alkaline water.

❖ About a half-hour after taking the prune juice, drink about 8-12 ounces of one of the juices you have chosen for the fast--juices such as apple, carrot, citrus, tomato, a combination of vegetable juices (vegetable juice is truly the best for cleansing), or a combination of green super foods and juice/water. If you are drinking fruit juice you may want to dilute it with part water to avoid too much sweetness and sugar. Make sure the juice you drink is organic. Fresh Vegetables or fruit juiced in your own kitchen are ideal.

❖ You will definitely want to have 2-3 "green drinks" daily during your cleanse. VITAMINERAL GREENS, AMAZING GRASS, GREEN MAGMA, or DR. TONY'S RADIANT GREENS are green super-food products that I use and recommend. Fresh wheat grass is a great addition to or supplementation for your green drinks. Another option for those who do not have unique health requirements is to take the green super-food drink in the morning and the straight wheat grass mid-day.

Kombucha Tea is a wonderful cleansing and alkalizing aid that suppresses the appetite. The tea will help your energy, nutrition levels, cleansing process and will assist in alkalizing your body. One 12 oz. bottle is best consumed in 4-6 oz. intervals throughout the day. This product can be found in most natural health food stores.

Alkaline Water can assist your body during the cleansing process, helping the body to remove excess toxins, fat build up and waste in the colon. Only drink this water for up to 2 weeks because you don't want to over-alkalize your body and create deficiencies from too much cleansing. Your body strives to be at a PH of about 7.36 and alkaline water generally has a PH of 8.5 to 10 which is why over-alkalizing could disrupt the balance of your body balance.

❖ Approximately 30 minutes after your juice, drink 12 or more ounces of alkaline water. You should be drinking 12 or more ounces of your selected juices every 2-3 hours. You can alternate juice one time and a super-food drink (made with alkaline water) the next time, or add some greens to every juice session. The green super foods create more satisfaction and satiation, delay hunger, provide energy, increase the rate of cleansing, and create more alkalinity in the blood (which is key to cleansing).

❖ Continue alternating juice and alkaline water every half-hour to an hour until you have consumed two quarts of juice. You can have more juice if you need it. I highly recommend drinking Kombucha tea throughout the day to aid in cleansing and satiation.

❖ Recommended: take 1 tablespoon of fresh-pressed flaxseed oil two to three times a day to aid in lubricating the bile and liver duct.

❖ On the fourth day, begin taking solids again. For the first couple of days try to eat only raw foods, then slowly add unprocessed cooked foods if desired.

The three-day cleanse two to four times a year will suffice (ideally at the beginning of each season), but a deeper and more thorough cleanse is sometimes needed, especially if a body has gone through many years of neglect. However, if you have never gone through a cleanse it is best to start with a three-day, and then advance to an eleven-day.

For example, if you are overweight, detoxifying from drug, alcohol, and nicotine addiction, or recovering from a battle with a disease in which your body has been subjected to consistent foreign substances such as pain killers, you would want to start with a couple three day cleanses to jump start the process of toxin elimination, and then advance slowly, perhaps adding days to work your body up to an eleven-day cleanse as your body's alkalinity has begun to balance. Always check with your physician before your cleanse if you have any unique health issues such as those listed above.

The longer eleven-day cleanse is different from the three-day because you start with a three-day juice cleanse, and then you have eight days of gradually adding raw foods and broths to your juice regime. The fiber that you are adding in the raw fruits and vegetable help to further push out the toxins that have been pulled from your organs into your bloodstream. A hot bath should be taken every night during your cleanse to aid the continual release of toxins.

The eleven-day cleanse can be used as a good general cleanser two or three times a year to reduce weight; when joints get stiff; to relieve constipation; for elimination of toxins. Those who are weak and feeble should not follow the plan for the full eleven days without supervision. The manner in which the foods are to be taken may be adjusted to suit your needs. Please refer to the next page for the steps for an eleven-day cleanse.

The Eleven-Day Cleanse

Day 1-3
❖ Follow the recommendation for the 3-Day Juice Cleanse conveyed above.

Day 4-5
❖ Eat whole fruits only. Use fruits such as grapes, melons, berries, tomatoes, pears, peaches, plums, apples, sulfur-free dried fruit such as prunes, figs and peaches.
❖ Soak dried fruits in water overnight, making them easier to digest.

Days 6-11
❖ Breakfast – Vegetable juice and/or green super-food drink
❖ Between breakfast and lunch have any kind of citrus fruits or berries
❖ Lunch - Salad of 3-6 vegetables and 2 cups of Essential Broth
❖ Between meals, drink plenty of alkaline water and vegetable juices as desired
❖ Dinner - 2 or 3 lightly steamed vegetables and 2 cups of Essential Broth
❖ Before retiring, drink vegetable or fruit juices if desired
❖ Eat plenty, but don't overeat

Recipe for Essential Broth

❖ 2 cups Carrot tops
❖ 2 cups Potato peelings ½" thick
❖ 2 cups Beet tops
❖ 2 cups Celery tops
❖ 3 cups Celery stalk
❖ 2 qts. water
❖ 1 Carrot & 1 Onion
❖ 10 Whole garlic cloves
❖ 1 Tbsp Miso paste
❖ Finely chop vegetables and slowly bring to a boil
❖ Simmer for about 20 minutes
❖ Strain out the vegetables, add the Miso, and drink the broth

Products to assist the cleansing process:

There are many different products that we use regularly or during a cleansing period and highly recommend. Some examples are:

- ❖ Digestive enzymes
- ❖ Kombucha Tea
- ❖ Green Matcha Tea
- ❖ Aloe Vera Juice
- ❖ Flaxseed meal and oil and Ground chia seeds
- ❖ Coconut oil
- ❖ Sea vegetables
- ❖ Green super-foods (such as wheat grass and spirulina)
- ❖ Chinese herbs and numerous other types of herbs

Please refer to the product recommendation guide on Page 115 for specific products to assist you in your cleanse.

Foods to Cleanse and Detoxify

Nature has provided whole foods which can help reverse illness and aid in cleansing and detoxifying. It is not necessary to spend fifty plus dollars on an intense cleansing kit or starve your body on only water and lemon juice for a month. There are various healing foods which you can easily incorporate onto the breakfast and dinner table and into lunch boxes for gradual cleansing. Let's take a look at some specific organs in our body and see which foods and beverages are natural healers and cleansers....

LIVER	KIDNEYS	STOMACH/COLON
Garlic, Seaweed, licorice root, turmeric, parsley, spinach, carrots, cucumber, celery, beets, cabbage, collards, kale, vitamin C rich produce (red bell peppers, tomatoes and citrus), cruciferous vegetables (broccoli, cauliflower and brussel sprouts), wild fish, and organic eggs and chicken	Seaweed, oily fish (salmon & sardines), raw olive oil, lemons, whole grains, dark leafy vegetables, apples, celery, raw nuts, beans & peas, cranberries, parsley, cilantro, rhubarb, raw milk and goat yogurt, miso, dandelion greens, apple cider vinegar, black cherries, apples, and apricots	Fiber (fresh fruit, vegetables, legumes and whole grains), figs, prunes, onions, chili peppers, rhubarb, cruciferous vegetables (cauliflower, broccoli, cabbage...), horseradish, filtered water, raw & sprouted nuts and seeds, whole & sprouted grains, sprouts, miso broth, ginger, fennel, leafy greens

THYROID (under active)	BRAIN	HEART
Seafood, as many raw & enzyme-rich foods as possible (sea weed/kelp, fresh vegetables and fruits , coconuts, coconut oil, coconut milk, flaxseeds, wild fish, only organic and free-range meats, carrots, spinach, apricots, asparagus, avocados, cucumbers, onions, squash, tomato, watermelon	Omega 3/DHA found in fish and flaxseed oil, blueberries, pumpkin seeds, almonds, apricots, bananas, beans, beets, black cherries, squash, dandelion greens, dates, eggs, figs, goat milk, leafy greens, lentils, parsley, walnuts, whole grains, natural olives	Yams, Bell Peppers, Omegas in Fish, Flaxseed, Coconut, and raw Olive oil, garlic, mushrooms, pumpkins (including the seeds and oil), apples, onions, avocados, green tea, sprouts, almonds, brazilnuts, cruciferous vegetables, walnuts, coconuts, whole grains, raw goat cheese and yogurt
SKIN	PANCREAS	
Miso, raw milk, goat yogurt, filtered water, raw & cold-pressed oils (coconut, olive, grapeseed, avocado, macadamia nut), avocados, raw nuts and seeds, wild fish (salmon), lots of raw veggies and fruits	Sweet fruits (apricots), tomatoes, root vegetables, organic vegetable juice, raw & cold-pressed oils, unrefined & whole salt (Celtic Sea Salt and Himalayan Sea Salt)	

Water and Proper Hydration

Why is hydration important to digestion?

Hydration through water, which by the way is naturally found in raw fruits and vegetables (raw vegetable juice is a great source of pure water), is important in helping to push the waste, insoluble fibers, and toxins through the body and digestive tract. It is recommended to drink about half of your body weight in ounces or more of water daily. Our bodies are 70% water, so this continual intake of pure water is essential to every bodily function. If you consume the necessary amount of pure water, the body will be more likely to hydrate and cleanse itself of daily toxins.

It is recommended that you need 70% of your food and liquid intake to consist of water-based foods and water, and not more than 30% from cooked foods. Raw fruits, vegetables, nuts, seeds, and sprouted grains are part of the 70% ratio of water sources needed for the body to live in an optimal balance. Raw fruits and vegetables are actually very high in water and the fiber in the food helps to transport the water to the cells and create hydration. My recommendation is to combine water and raw water-based foods to keep your body cleansed and hydrated from day to day.

Let's dive further...

Water is understandably a confusing and controversial topic. I am asked all the time to advise on which product or purification process is the healthiest. The challenge with water is that it is a local consideration in terms of assessing quality. Water quality will vary based on all kinds of variables such as the history of a locale's water system, how dense an urban area is, and the variety of water systems and products available. Fortunately, if you have access to the internet you can research the quality of water in your region and neighborhood, and then determine the steps you need to take in order to access drinking water that is as pure as possible.

Water is a necessity. To prove this, the body can survive 30+ days without food (although I don't recommend this), but can only last 3 days without water. So we are forced into a quandary of wanting to choose the cleanest product that will not break the bank while knowing that there might always be a better water source or system out there somewhere.

Most of the water not consumed out of the tap is purchased in plastic bottles of some type and size. The use of plastics in storing water is troublesome for three primary reasons. First, a half-billion units are sold per week. This adds tons of pollution to the already polluted environment. Second, many of the bottled water companies do not actually eliminate the chemical particles that define the water as impure, and there is very weak third party regulation to counter any claims of purity that bottled water brands list on their packaging. Lastly, a portion of plastic water bottles are made with BPA and other contaminants that potentially leach into the water and then your body, which of course is unsafe and dangerous to our health in the long run. So it is important to gradually eliminate the readily available low volume plastic water bottles, and ideally to invest in portable non-plastic containers for re-fill when on-the-go, and 3-5 gallon glass jugs to store and dispense water at home for daily use and emergency. This change-up will force manufacturers to start using safer containers, and using re-fill containers will also save you money in the long run.

My first criteria when choosing a water system is the filtration. Tap water provides millions of illegal harmful contaminants often including arsenic, radioactive drugs, sewage and potentially more invisible toxins so it is essential that we are all diligent to make sure our drinking and cooking water is as filtered as possible. A primary metric to use to measure the purity level of a water sample whether pre or post-filtered is the "TDS" level, which stands for "Total Dissolved Solids". TDS is the measurement of how many particles and contaminants are in the respective water. The basic rule is that the lower the number of TDS, the cleaner the water. I believe the average tap water has approximately 350 parts per million (ppm) of TDS. After reviewing examples of successful water filtration, I've learned that a successful TDS benchmark is 25. Any TDS count that falls within the ideal 0-25 TDS range is ideal.

As I said, the focal point of your investigation is to understand the systems and your local sources. I would need to write another book to examine all the local sources in the U.S. (rivers, lakes, springs, etc.), but I can get you started on the pros and cons of the most common systems that includes countertop filters, distillation, reverse osmosis and ionization. A system can be complex, and is naturally exaggerated by the seller so understanding the details and third party checking the systems is critical just as you would do your diligence for other major product purchases before you buy. The quality of any system depends on the filtration process so focus on the type and cost of the filters before you invest in a system.

Water Purification Systems

Countertop Filters can be a smart and safe way to go without spending a ton of money on a machine. I have asked water researchers/scientists what they feel is the best route to go and I have been told that a cost-effective route is to purchase a good home filter or distiller that attaches to your sink, run the water into a glass water holder and then add a portion of Himalayan salt to the water.

Distillation is essentially water that has been boiled, the particles and minerals have been separated and the vapor is then condensed to water. However, while distilled water is very clean the good minerals have been pulled out in the process so you want to add minerals back to the water once distilled. One such way that was recommended to me is to add ½ tsp of Himalayan Salt per 1 gallon of distilled water and your mineral content in the water will be restored. That could also be a good solution for those who have distilled water being delivered to their home.

Water Ionizers focus on alkalizing water which is fine for short term cleansing but not long-term. It is critical to know that water ionizers do not filter the water - you have to buy separate filters, which can add cost to an already costly system. Alkaline Water can assist your body during the cleansing process, helping the body to remove excess toxins, fat build up and waste in the colon. However, your body strives to be at a PH level of about 7.36 and alkaline water generally has a PH of 8.5 to 10, which is why drinking a high volume of alkaline water over multiple weeks will most likely disrupt your balance. I recommend only drinking high alkalinity water for up to 2 weeks when you need to cleanse, or if your doctor confirms you are very acidic, but I don't recommend this type of alkaline cleanse more than once per season (so about every 3 months.)

Reverse Osmosis machines purify/filter the water and remove particles and contaminants from the water leaving it clean but lacking in good minerals. If you have a RO machine I recommend also adding ½ tsp Himalaya salt per gallon to restore the minerals that have been lost. Many health food stores have RO systems set up so that customers can bring in their water containers, fill them up with the water and pay a low cost per gallon.

Another option is to find a natural spring near you where you can purchase "raw" spring water, and will know exactly what source it came from. Driving to a spring may not make sense depending on the distance to the location, but it is worth the time to log on to **www.findaspring.com** where you can enter your address and find the nearest spring source in your area that gives away or sells "raw" spring water. I've researched that raw spring water generally measures between 6.5 and 7.5 and sometimes even as low as 6.0. This is promising since that range is within the PH range that is optimal for human health. You also want to make sure you know the TDS number of the spring because, for example, a spring near a big city might contain many contaminants from local pollution.

CHAPTER
FOUR

MAKING THE TRANSITION

Establishing your Foundation for Change:
Make a Gradual and Measured Transition

We have introduced essential building blocks to begin building your foundation. Understanding the bodies' system of digestion is essential to getting started. Undergoing an initial cleanse to "clean the slate" will help start the process of breaking free of the binds that have prevented you from accessing the good energy that is waiting to be harnessed. This is all fundamental preparation for your transition.

There is no timetable for your transition. The results depend on your own will, passion, and unique lifestyle. It is non-linear and dictated solely by the paths you create. You will however, experience immediate results if you explore, discover, and empower yourself with the information in this guide. What I want you to understand is that your body took years upon years to reach its current state so you must be patient and always remember that these changes you are making are not just for a temporary period to prepare you for a night out. These changes are for a lifetime. The rate of change depends on what point you are starting from and how committed and consistent you are. Truly, I believe it depends on your passion. Passion is what drives us forward in all of our lives.

A gradual transition allows your body to systematically purge itself of accumulated waste materials, and helps you detoxify safely, without severe discomfort. The body and mind take approximately three to five weeks to adapt to each new change you make. So, you must separate your transition into parts, or what we more commonly think of as goals. One part is not necessarily more important than the next. For example, eliminating fried foods isn't more important than eliminating soda drinks or white flour. You will want to address each of these separately, yet in the context of your overall energy. Finally, you must set a realistic order. Each of us will struggle more with some parts, while others will hopefully come easier. Do not try to tackle every change at once, but start with one or a few at a time.

The basis of the transition I recommend is a gradual switch from a refined, processed, meat-based diet to a more natural, live, and plant-based diet. To help make the transition, we have created categories of substitutes and replacements to serve as guideposts along your transition.

When starting your transition, we have found that it is best to begin by examining the beverages you drink on a daily basis. The drinks we consume can be as damaging if not more damaging to our overall balance than foods can, and when combined with bad foods, they are adding toxicity to your body and mind at a damaging rate.

Transitioning to Functional Beverages

I. Highly Processed and Chemical Laden Beverages -- to be avoided if possible

Pasteurization means that beverages have been heated at a high degree to the point in which all the enzymes and most nutrients are killed. In addition, when a fruit is heated, the sugar is recognized as regular table sugar in your body.

- ❖ Tap Water
- ❖ Sodas and all sugar-sweetened drinks
- ❖ Sugar-Free and Diet Sodas
- ❖ Sport Drinks (that contain sugars, preservatives, food dyes, Sugar-free Substitutes)
- ❖ Chemical based Sugar-Free Substitutes (Aspartame, Nutrasweet, Splenda, Equal etc.)
- ❖ Coffee & Black Tea
- ❖ Alcohol (beer, all wine, sugary cocktails, liquor)
- ❖ Fruit Drinks/Juices with sugar and substitutes added
- ❖ Bottled and Pasteurized Juices (orange, apple, pineapple, grape, etc.)

II. Beverages high in anti-oxidants, minerals, energy -- moderate to freely

These beverages should be drunk in balance with pure water hydration, and are energy-lifting replacements for coffee, black tea, caffeinated and diet sodas:

- ❖ Green Tea & Matcha Green Tea
- ❖ Yerba Mate & Herbal Teas
- ❖ Red and White Tea
- ❖ Young Thai Coconut water
- ❖ Coconut Kefir
- ❖ High anti-oxidant berry juices (unsweetened and un-pasteurized if available)
- ❖ Pomegranate
- ❖ Cranberry
- ❖ Blueberry
- ❖ Goji berry
- ❖ Acai
- ❖ Raw Kombucha Tea
- ❖ Fresh fruit and organic vegetable juices (juiced fresh in a "juicer")

Recommendations on Natural Sweeteners:

STEVIA

A plant-based sweetener—can be bought in liquid or powder form at most natural foods stores. It has no sugar or fat, which means it cannot influence your blood glucose levels. It is also anti-fungal which means that it helps cleanse your blood. I use it to sweeten my teas, green drinks, and any beverage that needs to be sweetened.

YACON SYRUP

Yacon Root is a raw, low-calorie, low-sugar, molasses-like flavored syrup with a broad-spectrum nutrient profile. With special, natural fructoligosaccharide (FOS) sugars enables Yacon to be absorbed and used as a prebiotic or "food" in the digestive tract.

"Great for diabetics and sugar sensitivities, dieters, healthy diets, digestive imbalances, high cholesterol, and also aiding in athletic performance; making it an incredible, natural, top notch whole food and a sweetener to boot! It has been found and studied that *Yacon* syrup has very little influence on insulin spiking and is dramatically less glycemic-effect than sugar, honey, agave and/or maple syrup." (Darin Olien, Darin's Naturals)

Transitioning to Functional Whole Foods

When starting and continuing your transition, it is important that you always think of the foods you eat and the beverages you drink in terms of their energy value. In our fast paced lives, we are often placed into a variety of situations that require us to negotiate and accommodate our choices based on what is available at the time. Planning ahead is not always possible, and budget can be an issue. When transitioning to a good energy lifestyle, you will also go through adjustments in your financial priorities. If you have not started already, you will be shifting to natural and whole food grocers for your kitchen based food and beverages. Some of these foods are priced higher than the processed, refined, and bad energy foods at the traditional mass grocery chains. It is important to account for every dollar spent during this transition because it will help you to become a savvy shopper.

For instance, I realized that I could buy organic vegetables, fruits, nuts, legumes, etc. for a lesser price at the local farmers market, while I will purchase spices, seafood, unique product supplements and other specialty items at the larger natural food grocer. Also keep in mind that you will be buying less processed (pre-made) foods, soda and possibly less animal products (red meat, cheese, milk, butter, etc.), which will balance out the extra money spent on organic and natural foods. I will give you the guidelines you need to become an expert shopper in Chapter 18, but for now I want you to know that if your health is a priority, and you want to live a lifestyle full of zest, passion, and good energy, then you will find a way to adjust to the initial cost fluctuation.

All said, I guarantee that you will find that changing to a good energy lifestyle will actually cost you less in the long run, and as you move forward in your transition, you will see that it is saving you in the short run. One quick example is that you will find that you are making a lot more of your meals and beverages in your kitchen, and not depending on coffee shops and restaurants to feed you four to five days a week. Your doctor bills should hopefully diminish – healthy eating is truly a preventative practice. Really though, once you move further along, you will find that you enjoy investing in this new lifestyle because you cannot put a price on good health and good energy. Good energy is the common denominator for truly experiencing and enjoying our lives.

It is important not to get frustrated or feel overly guilty if you eat or drink something you know is not in the good energy category. Those emotions can cause as much damage as the food you are worrying about. Just the fact that you are aware of what you are putting into your body and how it affects you should empower you to believe that you can and will balance and adjust to any missteps in the future. There is no failure here. The concept of failure is bad energy, and I do not subscribe to it. I could not be creative and realize my potential if I take a huge step back each time I veer off my path. There is only the journey, and your transition will be one of continuous learning. Each misstep is a step forward.

The energy analysis breakdown below separates foods into categories that will help you as you begin to make choices on what foods to decrease, substitute, eliminate, and add during your transition:

Negative Energy Foods

I. Highly Refined Foods -- to be avoided whenever possible
Highly refined, processed, dead foods whose nutrients have been stripped through processing

- ❖ Any foods with artificial additives and preservatives
- ❖ Meats grown with hormones and chemicals
- ❖ Any dairy foods from animals raised on hormones and chemicals, or pasteurized
- ❖ Most canned foods
- ❖ Refined oils, especially hydrogenated oils
- ❖ Table salt
- ❖ Refined white or brown sugar
- ❖ Refined flours (white/unbleached flour)
- ❖ Refined grains, such as white rice

Low Energy Foods

II. Cooked or Slightly Processed Foods -- limit consumption
This group includes non-organic foods (except organic meat & dairy) that start off nutritionally sound but lose nutritional value through cooking or processing

- ❖ Baked chips
- ❖ Bottled, un-pasteurized juice (orange, apple, grape, pineapple, mango, papaya, etc.)
- ❖ All Wine
- ❖ Wheat and potatoes (specifically for those losing weight)
- ❖ Whole grain, non-organic cooked foods

❖ Non-organic cooked vegetables and fruits
❖ Non-organic frozen produce
❖ Non-organic spices and herbs
❖ Non-organic/organic dairy substitutes from soy and rice
❖ Non-organic vegetable and fruit juices
❖ Powdered and non-irradiated egg replacers, baking soda, baking powder
❖ Non-organic whole grain flours and grain products
❖ Free range, nitrite & nitrate free, and/or organic meats
❖ Processed sweeteners that aren't raw - maple syrup, maple sugar, agave, xylitol and date sugar

Moderate Energy Foods

III. **Organic and/or sprouted, cooked whole foods -- eat moderate amount**
These foods are all good energy choices, but are not the purest form of good energy.

❖ Whole grain organic flours and grain products
❖ Sprouted Breads
❖ Organic baked chips and tortillas
❖ Organic, sprouted, cooked whole grains (especially brown rice)
❖ Organic, soaked beans that are cooked
❖ Organic, raw, soaked nuts and seeds, cooked in sauces and dishes
❖ Jarred organic nut butters
❖ Organic whole foods and sauces bottled in jars
❖ Organic lead-free canned foods
❖ Organic raw sweeteners – raw honey and raw yacon syrup
❖ Organic dairy substitutes made from almond, hemp and other nut milks
❖ Raw organic dairy products
❖ Organic dried fruits
❖ Organic sprouted tofu (Wildwood)
❖ Organic, cold-pressed, grapeseed, macadamia nut and olive oil
❖ Fish, organic and/or wild
❖ Organic/free range eggs if desired
❖ Organic goat products (un-pasteurized if possible): milk, yogurt and cheese. (Goat milk is much easier for the body to digest than cow's milk because its mineral ratios are very similar to those in the human body)
❖ Nama Shoyu fermented soy sauce

High Energy Foods

IV. **Organic, sprouted or dried foods in their raw state -- eat freely**
These foods are great when added to your own home-processed foods:

- Sprouted, organic raw dips, spreads and sauces
- Organic, cold-pressed flaxseed, hempseed and coconut oil (raw/uncooked)
- Raw fats such as avocados
- Organic, raw, sprouted dried/dehydrated breads, crackers and cookies
- Fresh, organic vegetable and fruit juices
- Fresh, organic sprouted legumes, grains, nuts and seeds
- Organic spices and herbs, dried under 110 degrees temperature
- Sea vegetables
- Fresh, organic fruits and vegetables
- Tempeh
- Miso
- Kombucha Tea
- Raw organic coconut-based products like Coconut Aminos and Coconut Nectar
- Young Thai Coconuts – the coconut water is amazing for digestion
- Raw kefir
- Raw soups and smoothies
- Raw Cacao
- Green super-food blends, such as wheat grass and spirulina (organic and dried Under 115 degrees)

CHAPTER FIVE

EXERCISE: THE BEST FRIEND OF NUTRITION

In Chapter I, the Foundation, I challenged you to begin to think of your diet more in terms of the energy value rather than in calories. Likewise, I challenge you to think of exercise less in terms of losing weight, and more in terms of increasing your sustained and balanced energy. Losing weight the right way is just a fantastic byproduct of a good energy lifestyle.

To reach and maintain your overall optimum energy, it is essential to not only eat well, but also to maintain a consistent level of physical activity. Exercising your body brings a balance physically, emotionally and spiritually, and is thus a key to both vitality and rejuvenation. Studies have shown that exercising can reduce your biological age by 10 to 20 years.

Mind Shift

Drop all preconceptions about "working out" and "getting in shape", which are usually associated with weight loss. Exercise is a multifaceted tool. It plays a key role in all levels of detoxification through the simple but highly therapeutic process of sweating. It tones and improves the quality of your muscle tissue and stimulates the processes of digestion, metabolism and elimination. It also strengthens your lungs, heart and the activity of all organs. The circulation of the vascular and lymph systems is improved, resulting in better transfer of oxygen throughout the body. Regular physical activity can help protect your body from degenerative diseases, digestive disorders, cancer, osteoporosis, muscular dystrophy, obesity, menstrual irregularities, sexual dysfunction, and other health problems.

Individuality

Just as there is no <u>one</u> right diet, there is no <u>one</u> all purpose exercise program for everyone. However, the one factor that we all share is the need for exercise. As your eating habits change, so should your exercise abilities and motivation. Grab every ounce of energy and motivation and explore the world of physical activities. If you grow bored of exercise, maybe you haven't found your niche. Try looking outside of the gym. Outdoor activities such as hiking, walking in nature, surfing, tennis, biking, rollerblading and swimming are great forms of exercise and can be done with a friend. Yoga, Pilates, and dancing are amazing indoor activities that help mold your body into shape. The most important thing is to listen to your body. Don't push your body beyond its physical capability, but at the same time don't get lazy. Try to be active at least 4 times per week and break a sweat. Don't forget light resistance training (lifting light weights) for muscle toning and bone health. Remember that exercising consistently is critical if you want to see results!

Fitness and Metabolism are related

It is actually basic science and should be true for every person. The more muscle you have, the higher your metabolic rate, meaning that you will burn more calories at a resting rate. In short, muscle burns stored energy. Calories are measured in heat and are therefore stored energy, which is also equated with stored fat.

Energy is there to be used. If it is not used, it is generally stored as fat. Actual physical muscle helps burn calories or stored fat 24-7.

I am not talking about those large bulky muscles. Lean, compact muscles do the job. Building lean muscle through lifting light weights, or activities such as yoga, forces the body to use up more stored energy on a regular basis, aiding in fat elimination. As muscle replaces fat storages in the body, oxygen levels increase, energy increases, excess weight decreases, and the need for natural foods increase. When I say you have to eat to lose weight, I mean that if you starve yourself, then your body will metabolize your muscles, creating that flabby and soft look, and as we have just said, you need muscle to eliminate fat. Basically, muscle mass is a great tool that technically is working out for you all day even when you are sitting at a desk.

Exercise is therapeutic

We know that exercise will improve our muscle tone, strength, and circulation, but the therapeutic effect that physical activity has on the mind could be the most valuable gift we give ourselves each day. If you are one of the few people in the world with little to no stress, than you are in the extreme minority. Stress and anxiety can be just as harmful, if not worse, as smoking, drinking alcohol, and mowing down a cheeseburger, fries, and coke from a fast food joint. Making changes in your diet can certainly help you manage and even eliminate many stress sources, but in most cases the toxic buildup from stress needs a dual approach and that is where the best friend named "exercise" comes in. For example, you could be the healthiest eater at work, however, after staring at your computer for eight hours while being hounded by deadlines and various stress sources, your internal design is left in an acidic state.

Just as you are now planning ahead for your daily meals, you must plan ahead to exercise. Exercise helps to relax the body, increase blood flow (after sitting in a chair all day), release frustration and tension, and create happy endorphins. We tend to be overly mental and that bit of exercise allows your brain to let go and give in to peace. You don't need to exercise long and hard, which could create internal stress, but just enough to where you feel that tension release. Try to find a nice even balance between nutrition and exercise. The two will need to be working together in order to produce optimal good energy.

Exercise for the spirit

Exercising is critical for the body and mind, but we must also realize its potential to advance us spiritually. As I mentioned previously, exercise helps us escape that mental state that causes your head feel heavy. If your practice is meditation, reading, visualizing, or any other spiritual activity, you need to be in that relaxed state. Exercising prior to meditation does wonders for me. I can shake off the day, get my body relaxed, and turn off my brain. Now I am ready to exercise my spirit and forget about the day.

Eating for your workouts

When you start an exercise program, you will want to have an energy strategy to go with it. As we have said, every one of us has a unique body design, and therefore has different energy needs depending on the intensity, goals, and time of day of your workout. No matter what time of day, always follow the 'natural' versus 'processed' guide:

- ❖ Whole grains versus white flour and white rice
- ❖ Raw fats and oils versus fried and saturated oils
- ❖ Natural raw sugars instead of processed white sugar

On the following pages, I will give you general advice on the best way to energize for your workout depending on the time of day and the intensity.

There are general practices that all of us can follow when preparing the body for a workout. First, you need energy, and energy is created by what you put in your body so regardless of the time of day or intensity of workout, you will want to find the right energy source and should be conscious of how your body will channel that energy.

Morning Workout: Before and After
5 am – Noon

Your body is in a state of cleansing from about 4am until 8am. Naturally, your body will be emptier and more cleaned out in the morning than any other time of the day. This is a choice time to engage in physical activity because your body is not preoccupied with digesting a sum of food from the present day. The morning time is ideal for burning those extra stored sugars and fats—your body has less food to burn. I don't advise rolling out of bed, drinking some water and then doing one hour of intense cardio. Your body does need food-energy in some form. Keep it simple, high-energy and nutrient rich. Here are some examples of foods that I use for my morning energy demand:

❖ Green and/or Red super-food drinks made with water and chia seeds blended up
❖ Whole sprouted grains (sprouted bread (toast), whole grain/sugar-free cereal, brown rice, quinoa) or steel cut oats soaked in water over night; then cooked or eaten raw
❖ Dehydrated cookies or burgers
❖ Raw protein like almonds, walnuts or tempeh
❖ Small portion of fish or egg whites
❖ Vegetables or vegetable juice
❖ Starchy fruits like bananas and dates
❖ Young Thai Coconuts

Afternoon Workout
Noon – 5 pm

By the afternoon, you will have probably eaten 2-4 meals (hopefully smaller). If you are planning to work out in the afternoon, adapt your eating schedule so that you have the energy you need for an optimal exercise session. You should eat within the first 30 minutes after you awake, and then every few hours thereafter. A simple guideline is to eat something the size of your palm, about ½ hour prior to workout, depending on how quickly your body metabolizes food. Focus on the following whole foods and ingredients for sustained good energy:

❖ Dehydrated cookies or burgers
❖ Complex carbohydrates (whole grains such as brown rice, quinoa)
❖ Sandwich with whole grain or spouted bread, cashew mushroom burger, veggie or fish wrap with whole grain tortillas
❖ Lean animal or plant-based protein (fish, eggs, tempeh, sunflower seeds, almonds, walnuts, hempseeds, pumpkin seeds)
❖ Raw fats (avocado, raw nuts, olive oil, and especially coconut oil)
❖ Berries or other raw fruits
❖ Salad (vegetables, tempeh, chia seeds, fish, nuts and seeds, olive oil, balsamic vinegar, avocado, sunflower dressing)
❖ A second green/red super-food drink. Or make a smoothie and add a scoop of the green or red super-food powders and 1 Tbsp Chia seeds

Evening Workout
5 pm – 10 pm

It is always challenging to work out in the evening due to a lack of energy, exhaustion after a full work day, or the desire for a big heavy dinner. My recommendations are very similar to the eating habits for an afternoon workout. First, eat a variety of small meals that include whole foods in their natural state every 2-4 hours throughout the day. This will help you keep your energy level up, and help keep you motivated for your workout. Secondly, if you plan to exercise after 6 pm, I advise eating a small good energy meal by 5:30 or 5:45. Here are some examples of quick energy meals to revitalize the body for evening exercise:

❖ Dehydrated cookies and burgers full of complex carbohydrates, protein and raw fats
❖ A small piece of salmon and a handful of baby carrots
❖ A slice of sprouted bread with nut butter or coconut oil and honey
❖ Chia seeds added to a smoothie or green drink (chia seeds give endurance)

After your workout, I wouldn't advise eating a big meal. Keep it simple and light, such as fish and vegetables, soup, brown rice and vegetables, salad with sprouted bread and avocado.

Digestion and Exercise
The rule of thumb is to give your body a half-hour to an hour between eating or working out. The time taken is determined by the intensity of your planned workout and what you ate. The digestion of food takes a great deal of energy from your body. Exercise also requires energy. I don't advise eating and exercising simultaneously or within 15 minutes of each other. Let your body digest a bit and then use that energy, which is now filtering throughout your body, for exercise. Raw foods will generally go through your system quicker, about 15-30 minutes. If you have eaten a lot of animal products, give your body at least 30 minutes before engaging in exercise. You can have a green drink 10 minutes before exercising and it should give you great energy.

Low intensity exercises require less pre-digestion time than high intensity. For example, if you are going for a walk, you probably only need about 15 minutes for proper digestion. If you are going to do yoga, aerobics, weight lifting, jogging, or anything that is moderate to high intensity and increases your heart rate above normal, then you want to wait at least 30 minutes.

There are foods and drinks designed for energy boosts while you are exercising. They do not require resting periods for digestion. Some great examples are:

- ❖ Young Coconut water – highest in electrolytes
- ❖ Dehydrated Energy Bars
- ❖ Dehydrated crackers and burgers
- ❖ Sprouted dehydrated nuts and seeds
- ❖ Raw trail mix (dried fruits, raw nuts, and seeds)
- ❖ Raw, Coldpressed Coconut Oil
- ❖ Organic Fruits of Choice (dates and bananas are best)
- ❖ Organic vegetables (carrot sticks are best)
- ❖ Kombucha Tea
- ❖ Energy bars (look for raw, dehydrated, uncooked, no regular or artificial sugars)

Tips on Protein Drinks

- ❖ Protein Drinks are popular, and are better drunk before or after the workout, not during. Try to allow 15 minutes before working out after you have a protein drink. Ideally stick to hemp protein and rice protein.

- ❖ Whey protein is fine for building muscle faster if that is your goal, but stick to products that are pure whey without preservatives, artificial sweeteners, and ideally brands that are organic or hormone-free.

- ❖ Avoid isolated soy protein because it is so processed and toxic that you are better off eating animal protein. See Chapter 10 for more on soy and isolated soy protein.

For those with fast metabolisms

For those of you who digest and burn food very quickly, you may need to eat a larger quantity prior to a workout, and/or bring food for a mid-workout snack. If your blood sugar drops quickly when you exercise, you should pay attention and plan ahead. Eat more complex grains, good fats and lean protein before exercising. Fat provides the body with longer lasting energy, so load up on the almonds, salmon and good raw oils. One tablespoon of raw coconut oil right before a workout has produced amazing results for my family. Coconut oil is raw and un-storable so it circulates energy continuously.

After a workout

Be kind to your body after exercising. It needs to repair and re-hydrate. Drink lots of clean filtered water; eat some lean protein such as:

- ❖ Fish, tempeh, eggs, raw nuts (almonds, pumpkin seeds, hemp seeds, walnuts)
- ❖ Healthy raw fats such as avocados, coconut oil, flaxseed oil, raw nuts; whole grain breads; grains such as quinoa (extremely high in protein) and brown rice
- ❖ Vegetables, especially greens
- ❖ Easily digested protein drinks (hemp protein, rice, or nut based)
- ❖ Fresh fruit eaten by itself.

It is also beneficial to take a good quality calcium/magnesium (see chapter 16 for specifics) after exercising to help relax the muscles and prevent cramping and soreness the next day. The following products can be great for repairing muscles and joints (see chapter 16).

- ❖ MSM,
- ❖ Turmeric
- ❖ Protein enzymes
- ❖ Raw omega fatty acids
- ❖ Ginger
- ❖ Blue-Green algae ('Blue Mana")

Supplemental Products for more energy
There are various food-based products which aid in energy and endurance.
My choices are:

- ❖ Cordyceps mushroom
- ❖ Schizandra Berry, Acai Berry
- ❖ Spirulina, Blue-Green algae, Wheat Grass and other greens
- ❖ Matcha Green Tea (See chapter 16 for more information)

Maca root is another useful herb for sustained energy without the caffeine. Maca has been used by ancient cultures for thousands of years for energy, hormone balancing, focus, stamina, and much more. I encourage you to research these food-based supplements, and see what works best for you.

Advice for the body builder
Most body-builders believe they **must** eat meat in order to build muscle, Wrong! It is the amino acids, which make protein that our bodies need. Amino acids are not only found in animal protein, but they can be found in whole grains, nuts, seeds, and legumes (especially tempeh), sea vegetables, sprouts and vegetables; some of which are complete proteins. Body builders who have relied on an animal protein diet find that once they stop exercising they tend to lose muscle tone quickly. However, those who build muscle on a more plant-based protein diet will sustain their muscle mass better.

So exercise is the keystone while nutrition is the cornerstone or something like that. The two play off the other like all great acts essentially generating good energy for the body, mind, and spirit. One however cannot get the most out of exercise if they are not correctly balancing your energy through the right fuel. Actually, if you told me that you are so busy during the week that you didn't have time to eat right, but you had time to exercise three days, I would have to tell you that you have it backwards. Nutrition leads the way because without it, you will not have the energy you need to advance your exercise program. Yours will be a cart without a horse, and your program will become one of frustration in which you see very little change. You will be more prone to giving up or cutting back to the point where exercise becomes a survival technique rather than a consistent part of your daily schedule.

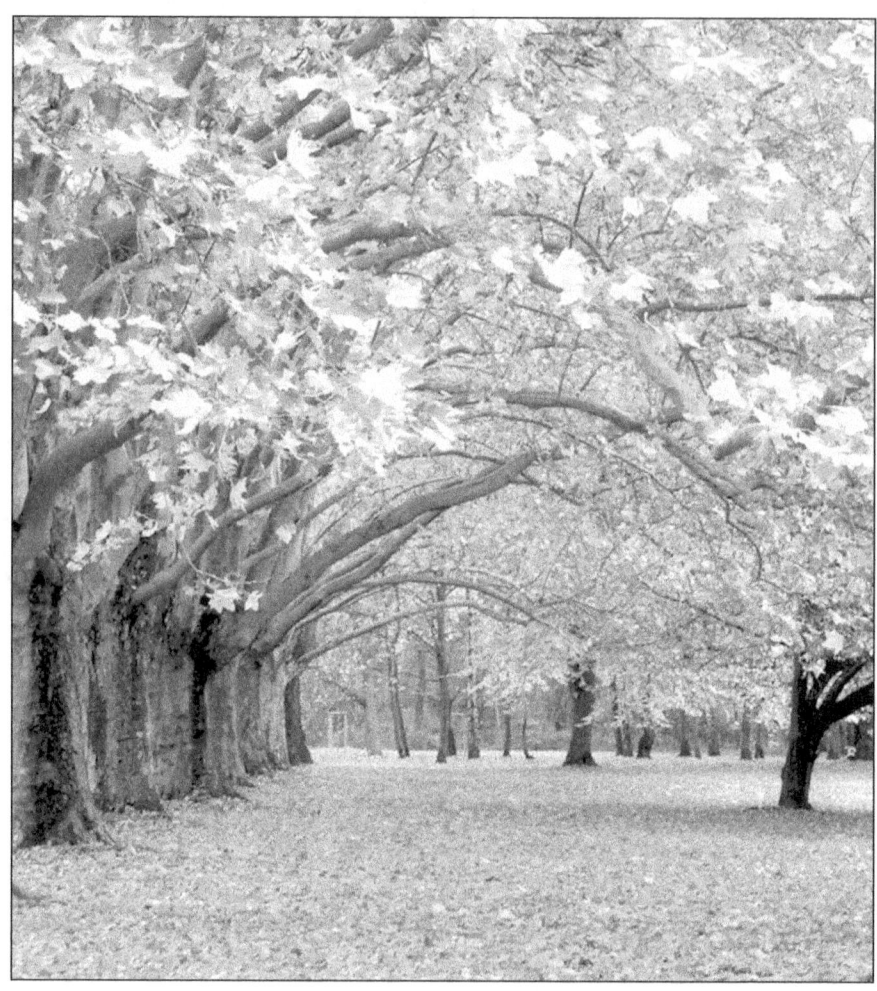

"In Order to change we must be sick and tired of
being sick and tired" ~ Author Unknown

CHAPTER
SIX

EXERCISING THE SPIRIT

What creation does a balanced diet have on the growth and clarity of our spirit?

Men and women throughout history, when striving for spiritual perception and clarity, have gravitated to a raw, plant-based diet. By contrast, stimulating foods such as meats, dairy and processed foods as well as beverages containing sugar, caffeine and alcohol require excess energy to break down—leaving the body overworked and tired. Try eating a heavy cooked meal and see if you are able to focus or meditate for a long period of time. Because you have fueled with such hard-to-digest foods, you will most likely lose clarity, and have a desire to go into a sort of mental hibernation. These heavy foods have a dampening influence on your mind and spirit. Discernment and clarity are almost always compromised until the foods are thoroughly digested in your system. If your energy is low due to the intake of negative to low energy foods, the byproduct can be a subtle impatience that causes frustration. Frustration is a pre-requisite to anger, which is a primary for stress. Stress places blocks around your spirit, preventing you from accessing the center of your being. One's internal compass can break. The result can be a general or succinct loss of direction. Some prefer to it as becoming ungrounded. I prefer to it as another example of being out of the moment and out of balance. This precipitous imbalance that begins with how one is fueling causes the body to reciprocate into a fight or flight mode, generally responding to your negativity by creating acid. The body then must create fat cells and plaque to absorb this toxic acid and neutralize it so that the acid doesn't harm your organs, veins, arteries, and your whole system.

This imbalance I defined is an example of the way our health must always be viewed and examined through a holistic lens. Eating bad food can create the bad energy. Your mind reacts by producing negative emotions, which in turn gives you distressed focus and mental clarity, which in turn shuts down your spiritual awareness. The cycle is a vicious one, in which your mind will learn to react to negative events or outside stresses by demanding food that is associated with pleasure. If you've always been eating low to negative energy foods such as cheeseburgers, French fries, sugary sodas, and other fried, dead, and processed foods, your body will actually demand more of them, which only creates more impatience, frustration, and a reduction to total depletion of good sustained energy. You could be the most spiritually committed person in your family, but if your diet and exercise are not in balance, you will find that exercising your spirit is
an extreme challenge, and that a muddled awareness is the end result.

We might ask how we can teach ourselves to break the cycle of turning to negative to low energy foods that we have been eating since we were children.

The first step is to learn to recognize the panic mode button when it triggers your body to demand a pleasure balance to the negative stress. This is where we must teach ourselves to be able to exercise our spirit on the run. We must turn to the spirit in those moments of mental stress, which are often predictable, and use the spirit to cut the stress off at the passing. When you are in a panic or stress mode, try taking deep breathes and clear your mind. If you can slow your breathing down to 10 breaths per minute, you can eliminate various stresses and emotions, and gain the temporary focus to make a good energy choice. This is the point where it is crucial to have good energy foods readily available. This is easier when you are at home, and have your kitchen, but this becomes challenging if you are in an office, car, airport, or on the go. Train yourself to have portable and functional foods with you at all times. You will learn strategies for eating in balance when you are away from home in the following chapter.

Once you catch your breath and gain your focus, and clarify the cause of your craving for pleasure, find the good energy foods that you have readily available, take a few bites, and discover how the process will create a new and much healthier cycle to replace the old one. Your mind will now associate good energy foods as being a solution for stress and negativity. You will now be in a cycle towards a more healthy body, which will enable you to be more aware of your spirit, even when you are not in the comfort of your home. Learn to make your body a willing and able tool to help you during this transition to greater energy on every level. Start out by practicing your own method of calming yourself before you start eating.

Through wise eating, you may help yourself in times of conflict and spiritual deprivation. Many people who are reaching for a higher level of living believe that foods only reduce access to the spirit. I believe there are fundamental elements of truth in the practice of cleansing the body of internal influences created by foods, but also believe that we should find a balance of allowing our spiritual awareness to guide the body to recognize and associate good energy foods with more access. Through occasional cleansing and juice fasting, your mental and spiritual perception can be made very sharp. The process of transitioning, cleansing, and occasional fasting teaches you to listen to your body, so that you only eat what your body needs and therefore craves, rather than overeating and consuming foods that have very little function at all for your energy or overall health. Don't work against yourself by indulging in those very foods, drinks and emotional drama, which are going to cross out all the efforts toward seeking the objectives of your spirit, body and mind.

Our body and mind cannot be in total balance without an ability to access our spirit. The spirit teaches us to stop, cleanse the mind, and discover the truth that is inherent within each of us. We can still operate with good energy on the physical and mental planes of our existence, but we will raise our awareness, understanding, and atonement if we are able to press pause on the false reality, and discover our path.

CHAPTER
SEVEN

Planning Ahead for your Energy Demand

Perhaps the most difficult and adjustable balance to establish during your transition is making the time to consistently prepare the meals for you and your family in your own kitchen. While this may be difficult in the beginning of your transition, the results are immediate.

Over the last ten years, I have fine-tuned a strategy for myself and family that give us sustained energy throughout our entire day-span, and literally transformed our health and overall lifestyles. We call it the "Drink plus Five". This is not a program or one-size-fits-all plan. Think of it as a set of flexible parameters that will help you create a custom diet that suits your energy demand.

Five plus one

Meal time is generally broken down into four categories across the world: Breakfast, Lunch, Dinner, and a hodgepodge of snacks depending on what are available. The problem with the three major meals per day routine is that it is both rigid and unrealistic for the pace of today's lifestyle schedules and energy demand. If more than three to four hours subside between meals, your energy drops, and your hunger may start to control your mind and therefore your body.

Most of us awake between the hours of 6 and 8am. The first energy of your day might be a bowl of cereal, muffin, or croissant and some coffee or tea, or in extreme cases, just coffee. This means that five hours may pass before your next feeding. This is too long. Your body at this point is starving for energy and is most likely slipping into an acidic state. By 11am, you may start to lose control over the decision making process, and you might gain the single all encompassing urge to satisfy your hunger and provide comfort for the initial stress you are feeling from your day. The choice you make can be driven by this overwhelming emotion, and the only way to make a good energy decision is if you have planned ahead. Planning ahead is the solution. If you have planned ahead, you will have good energy foods that you have already prepared so that you do not reach the extreme point, which could be emotional hunger or a drop in your blood sugar level, when you no longer care how you satisfy your hunger and need for energy.

Wake up on purpose

Let's first go back to the beginning of your day when you first awake. This is a crucial time because your body is an overall cleansing phase. It is void of nutrients and probably dehydrated from 6-10 hours without water. Your stomach is empty and just waiting for vital nutrients and life giving enzymes. This is also a crucial time because you want to detoxify your body from the preceding day, and start fresh. I have evolved a beverage ritual that both detoxifies my body, and then fills it with every nutrient it needs for the coming day. I start every day with this beverage sequence that helps jumpstart me out of bed; a blend of energy so vital to my need for nutrients, and overall energy demand that I rarely have a problem with waking up with a purpose, even during a challenging week of 12-16 hour day-spans.

The highlight of my day is the precious "Green Drink". It is such a crucial step towards a new lifestyle. If you were to commit to just one element out of the entire road map I have provided, it would be the daily green drink. Dr. Tony O'Donnell, creator of VIBRANT GREENS, says that,

"Super-foods are a concentrated potent source of vitamins, minerals, enzymes, antioxidants, fiber and the essential amino acids, which reputedly add alkalinity to our system, balance us, increase our energy, improve stamina, sharpen mental activity, and deodorize and cleanse the cells and colon. Super-foods are a return to the basics of the food chain."

Super-foods are my favorite energy drinks that I combine throughout the morning as I start my day. I actually start with the red super-food drink, wait 15 minutes, then move on to the green super-food drink, and then usually make a tea to go with my first meal of the day.

Red Super-food Drink
- ❖ Prepare and drink upon waking up
- ❖ Water mixed with 1 scoop of DR. TONY'S POMEGRANATE POWDER or CATIE'S VITAMIN C powder, mixed with water
- ❖ Antioxidant rich berries, packed w/absorbable Vitamin C, Potassium and minerals
- ❖ Another option is to purchase a green super-food blend that already has the berries added such as Goji, Acai, etc. Amazing Grass makes such a product in either their traditional super-food blend or Amazing Meal which also has hemp protein added.

Green Super-food Drink
- ❖ Green Super-foods blend
- ❖ Wheat Grass
- ❖ Green grasses, Sea vegetables, Spirulina, Blue-Green Algae
- ❖ Detoxifying, cleansing, alkalizing, nutrient-rich
- ❖ High in omega fatty acids, fiber, amino acids, and packed with energy
- ❖ Sweeten with Stevia, Yacon Syrup, Cinnamon and/or Vanilla

Herbal Tea
- ❖ Yerba Matte
- ❖ Green Tea, Matcha Green Tea
- ❖ Sweeten with Stevia, Yacon Syrup, Cinnamon and/or Vanilla
- ❖ Kombucha Tea

Morning Supplements
This is also a great time to plan your vitamin, mineral, and/or herbal supplements for the day. Many supplements are best taken with food, so I would recommend putting them into a small baggie that you could take throughout your day with the various meals.

Energy Meal One – Breakfast

Your body has now just received a complete blend of nutrients to blast you off into your busy day. This is a great time to make a small meal before you leave the home, and also an ideal time to prepare your lunchbox, (that's right, I said lunchbox), for your time away from home. I'll get to the lunchbox, but let's talk about this first meal of your day. The drink has given you nourishment and jumpstarted your metabolism. Now, your body needs sustenance or dense energy. There was a time in my life when I would only eat fruit from the time I awoke until my next meal. I found that I had to negotiate with a decline in blood sugar, which resulted in a rapid decrease in energy and mental focus. I do not advocate eating only fruit until your next meal because the excess sugar can create too much acid and could make your blood sugar drop too quickly.

Wait 15-30 minutes before eating a more substantial breakfast, such as:
- ❖ Sprouted, cooked or raw grains/nuts/seeds with raw sauces and sweeteners
- ❖ Whole grain cereal with non-dairy milk (hemp or almond)
- ❖ Cream of brown rice or buckwheat with raw honey or yacon syrup, cinnamon and almond milk and 10-12 soaked walnuts or almonds
- ❖ Whole grain waffles (no dairy/hydrogenated oil) with berries and 1 tsp raw maple syrup and coconut oil
- ❖ Cooked brown rice or steel cut oats (soaked 1st) with raw honey, cinnamon and almond milk
- ❖ Animal protein such as fish or poultry with sprouted bread
- ❖ 1 egg with 1/3 cup egg white, veggies & goat cheese
- ❖ Coconut or goat yogurt with flaxseed meal and granola and a handful of raw almonds
- ❖ Sprouted bread with nut butter and an apple
- ❖ Salad/protein wraps in a whole grain tortilla

Those are just some ideas. Be creative and see what works best for you. If you want to have fruit in the morning, you are better off eating the proteins, fats and carbohydrates recommended previously and then wait at least an hour to eat fruit. Remember, if your body is trying to digest a large breakfast, energy is drawn to that function, leaving little leftover for brainpower or physical work so eat in moderate portions, and consider enzyme supplements.

There will be days when you just don't have time to eat a breakfast meal between your drinks and arriving at your job or whatever your schedule requires. If you don't have time for breakfast, then here are few quick solutions that will keep you focused mentally, and will provide energy for any type of physical activity:

These are easily digested foods that give you quick energy. They are also great snacks for energy boost, and are very portable for easy store and transport.

- ❖ Munching on natural, simple/complex carbohydrates such as fresh and dried fruits with raw almonds.
- ❖ Vegetable juice smoothie with green super-foods and Matcha Green Tea added
- ❖ <u>Soaked</u> nuts, <u>dehydrated</u> sprouted breads, crackers and cookies

Energy Meals Two-Four: 11am – 7pm

Let's go back to preparing your lunchbox. Leaving home without a pack of food is a risk, not only for your health, but it is just bad practice. The world is an unpredictable place. It is better that you are self-sufficient incase variables arise that prevent other people from feeding you. Depending on your time, it is often easiest to prepare your lunch the night before, or at least plan it out so that you are ready in the morning. This pack or lunchbox should consist of the three meals you will need every 2-4 hours from the time you leave your home to the time you return.

Our definition of a meal is not that which has multiple courses. A meal can be anything you want it to be, but it has a function. It can be as simple as an apple and a small handful of almonds, 6 rice crackers dipped in humus, or a handful of baby carrots. A meal's function is not only to fulfill you, but also to energize you for the next few hours. If the meal is too big, then your body will have to expend all its energy digesting it. Enzyme supplements can help if you overeat, but this is not the answer. The solution is to pack your lunchbox with moderate but satisfying food portions that are tasty to satisfy you emotionally, and full of nutrients to continually recharge your battery until you are home.

Late Morning and Afternoon Snack Options:

- ❖ 1 spelt tortilla or sprouted whole grain tortilla with 2 Tbsp humus
- ❖ Carrots, red bell pepper & cucumber dipped in sunflower dressing/dip
- ❖ 1 apple and 2-3 dehydrated cookies
- ❖ Half of a natural, raw bar (Amazing Grass or Green's Plus Bar, Lara Bar, Revolution dehydrated bars, etc.) with a handful of soaked walnuts or almonds
- ❖ Apple with 2 tbsp peanut butter
- ❖ A dehydrated cracker or chips
- ❖ Piece of fruit or ½ cup of berries with some soaked almonds
- ❖ Non-dairy yogurt
- ❖ Soaked nuts with dates
- ❖ Young Thai Coconut
- ❖ Kombucha Tea
- ❖ Whole grain crackers dipped in nut pate

Salads with raw dressings are good raw choices for lunch. If you choose to eat cooked foods, such as whole grains, legumes, veggies or fish and other meats, eat them after eating raw foods. Cooked foods have lost all their enzymes to aid digestion so they will hold up the digestion and assimilation of the raw foods that you ate prior. Furthermore, cooked foods can ferment -- causing uncomfortable and embarrassing gas. Finally, raw vegetables and juices are great portable replacements when you don't have time to stop.

Here are some tasty and good energy lunch ideas:

- Pita bread stuffed with nut pate, crumbled tempeh or slices of fish or chicken, avocado, lettuce, tomato, and non-dairy dressing
- Large salad with tuna salad (made with veganaise), chopped veggies, goat feta, and vinaigrette dressing and an apple
- Lettuce or collard greens wraps filled with spread (almond pate, humus or almond dressing), grilled fish strips, and veggies of choice
- Lettuce wraps filled with finely chopped grilled veggies, sautéed in Asian-style marinade.
- Sandwich made with sprouted bread, natural veggie burger, dehydrated grain burgers, or grilled fish/turkey, goat cheese, avocado, dressing, tomato and sprouts
- 1-2 corn tortillas with goat, sheep or rice cheese; black beans, veggies, salsa, avocado, and lettuce
- Non-dairy soup with whole grain or sprouted crackers and dip
- Sushi rolls – try to find rolls made with brown rice and without mayonnaise
- Tuna Salad sandwich (made with Veganaise), topped with fresh veggies
- Brown rice or lean white meat with stir fried veggies
- Quinoa Tabouli with small salad
- Quinoa salad (cooked quinoa with olive oil, cilantro, Celtic Sea Salt, black beans, corn, red bell pepper, and a tsp of Veganaise)

I recommend always taking at least fifteen minutes to stop and find a relaxing, comfortable space, where you can meditate, chew, and enjoy your food at an even pace. Relaxation while eating will also aid in proper digestion.

Energy Meal Five: Early Dinner

By dinner time, you should not be famished. Most of our energy demand occurs between 7a and 6p so you should have consumed 80-85% of your daily intake by then. Dinner should not be heavy, loaded with cooked carbohydrates. Keep it simple with lots of veggies, light protein and healthy fats. Dinner should be concluded by 7 or 7:30 p.m. Remember to eat your raw foods before your cooked foods. Relax, breathe, chew, and enjoy!

Dinner Options:

- ❖ Fish or chicken strips stir fried with veggies in teriyaki sauce
- ❖ Lg. Asian Salad (Thai tofu, sesame seeds, snow peas, red pepper, butter lettuce and/or napa cabbage, tomatoes, and Asian dressing 4 oz.
- ❖ Grilled Salmon, steamed broccoli & cauliflower with Coconut Aminos or Tamari and seasonings
- ❖ Spelt or quinoa pasta with marinara or "Pesto" sauce, with grilled veggies on top
- ❖ Shrimp & veggie stir-fry with butternut squash
- ❖ Baked butternut squash with coconut oil, cilantro, lime juice, Celtic Sea Salt and spices
- ❖ Ahi or Squash Taquitos
- ❖ Non-dairy soup with a salad or cooked whole grain
- ❖ Halibut, Ahi or Salmon with veggie Kabobs
- ❖ Tostada/Taco Bar (corn tortillas, goat/rice cheese; black beans or tempeh, veggies, salsa, guacamole, lettuce, olives
- ❖ Curry-coconut quinoa
- ❖ Grilled veggie and fish in lettuce wraps
- ❖ Breakfast: Quiche or Spinach Egg Frittata
- ❖ Large salad topped with protein, whole grains, veggies and non-dairy dressing
- ❖ See the recipe section of the Just Good Energy website for more dinner ideas

Tip on Late Evening Snack

After 8:00 PM, if you need a snack, it is best to eat simple, easily digested foods, such as:

- ❖ Fruit and raw fruit sauces
- ❖ Smoothies
- ❖ Raw or dehydrated desserts/snacks
- ❖ Air Popped Popcorn
- ❖ Dates and soaked almonds
- ❖ Young Thai Coconut

Making time for a good energy lifestyle

Time is a formidable obstacle during the transition to a healthier lifestyle. My advice is to learn how to use time to your advantage. The time you take to prepare your own meals for your day will pay off in the short and long run. You will become more efficient as your good energy foods are readily available throughout your day. You won't constantly be wondering where you are going to get your next meal, and you will have absolute control as the gatekeeper to your health.

Sample 7 Day Menu

	1st Thing	Breakfast	Snack	Lunch	Snack	Dinner	Snack
Day 1	"Red Drink" and then the "Green Super-food Drink"	1-2 Slices sprouted/whole grain bread w/ natural nut butter & apple butter & 1 apple	carrots, red pepper & cuc w/ 2-3 Tbsp natural humus	Salad: 2-3 cups lettuce, sprouts, tomatoes, 1 oz. goat cheese, 2 oz. free-range chicken, tofu or tuna & vinaigrette	1 piece of fruit and a handful of raw and/or soaked almonds	4 oz. Salmon, sautéed veggies w/ Tamari, Coconut/ Grapeseed oil & seasonings	2 cups popcorn - ideally air popped or made with grapeseed or coconut oil, use Sea Salt
Day 2	"Red Drink" and then the "Green Super-food Drink"	3/4 cup cooked brown rice (soaked 1st) w/ honey, cinnamon & almond milk	1 piece of fruit and small handful of raw and/or soaked walnuts	1-2 corn tortillas & goat/soy/rice cheese; black beans or tempeh, veggies, salsa, avocado, lettuce	Naturally sweetened yogurt: soy, goat or cow	shrimp & veggie stir-fry w/ baked butternut squash	coconut date roll w/ 5-10 soaked almonds hot tea
Day 3	"Red Drink" and then the "Green Super-food Drink"	1/3-1/2 cup egg whites or 2 whole eggs, veggies & goat cheese	raw food bar: Vegan Bar, Lara Bar, Raw Bar or healthy cooked granola bar	tuna salad, 1 cup lettuce, veggies, & my healthy thousand Island dressing & 1 apple	small bowl fruit salad with coconut & natural granola	Dairy-free, Veg-based soup, 1/2 cup brown rice or curry/coconut quinoa	sliced fruit dipped in my raw peaches n' cream sauce
Day 4	"Red Drink" and then the "Green Super-food Drink"	Naturally sweetened Soy Yogurt w/ 1/3 cup natural granola	1 cup of Apple Waldorf Salad - dairy free	2-3 lettuce or nori wraps (nut pate, grilled veggies, guacamole)	1/2 of a peanut butter and jelly sandwich on sprouted/whole grain bread	spelt/quinoa pasta (3/4 cup) w/ non-dairy sauce, steamed veggies & 4 oz. of fish/ chicken	1/2 cup Coconut Milk ice cream (Coconut Bliss or So Delicious)
Day 5	"Red Drink" and then the "Green Super-food Drink"	1 egg w/ 1/3 cup egg white, veggies & goat cheese on a piece of sprouted/ whole grain bread	apple slices dipped in 1-2 Tbsp of peanut or almond butter	veggie stir-fry w/ fish in a spelt or corn tortilla	handful of raw/soaked almonds or walnuts and a date	Lg. Salad (chicken, almonds, snow peas, red pepper....Chinese dressing	popcorn
Day 6	"Red Drink" and then the "Green Super-food Drink"	1 cup apple waldorf salad or fruit salad with raw almonds	1 spelt tortilla w/ 2 Tbsp humus	sandwich with sprouted bread w/ lean chicken/tuna, & veggie toppings	sliced veggies dipped in my sunflower/ almond dressing	ahi & veggie kabobs & small salad w/ dressing of choice	piece of fruit
Day 7	"Red Drink" and then the "Green Super-food Drink"	1 cup hot cereal: cream of brown rice or wheat, oatmeal or other grain with honey & raisins	1/2 of a raw bar	1 cup Brazilian Potato Stew w/ a small salad	apple & 1-2 tbsp peanut or almond butter	Black bean tostada (1 corn tortilla, 1/3 c beans, veggies, salsa, etc.	Berries & soaked almonds (10)

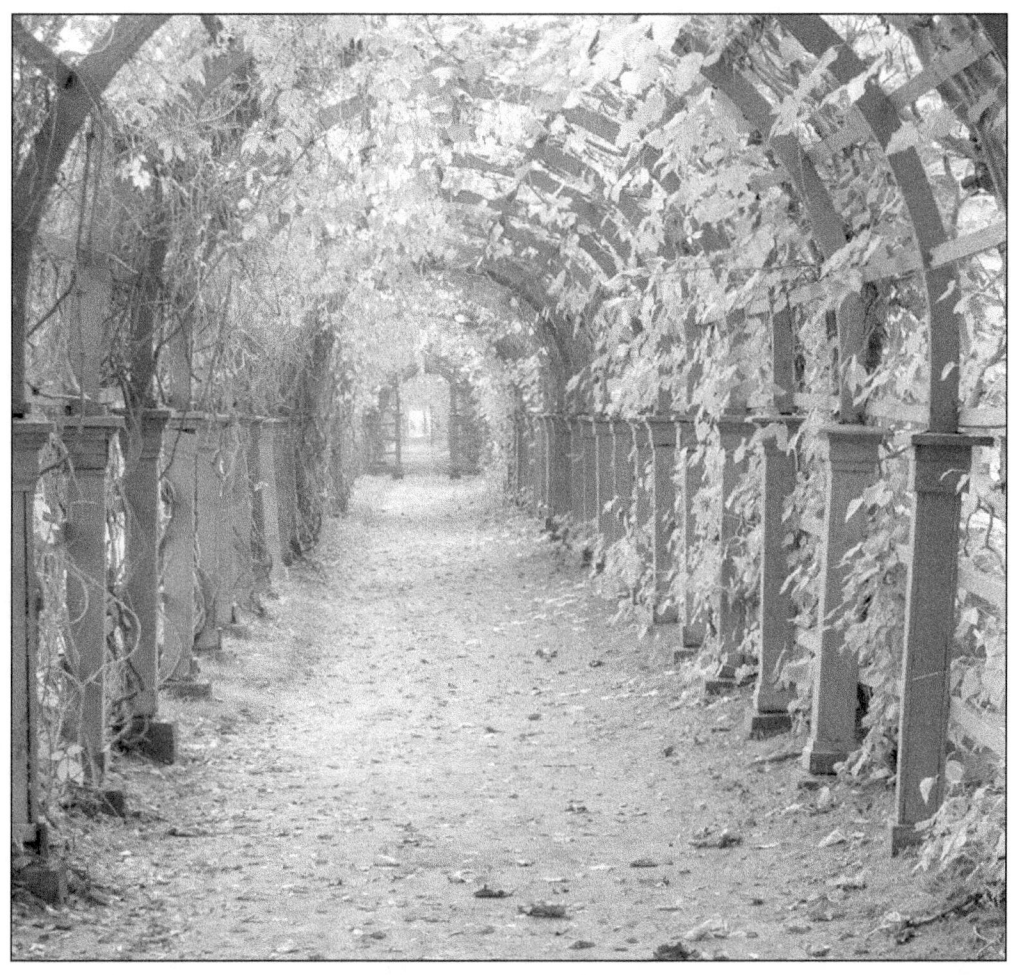

"The doctor of the future will give no medication, but will interest his patients in the care of the human frame, diet and in the cause and prevention of disease."
~ Thomas Edison

PART II

FOODS AND HOW THEY AFFECT THE BODY

Chapter 8
Fats and Oils – The Essential Balance

Chapter 9
Raw, Fermented, Dehydrated, and Super Foods

Chapter 10
Processed Foods

Chapter 11
Animal Products

Chapter 12
Basic Food Combining

Chapter 13
Acid Vs. Alkaline

Acid/Alkaline Food Chart

Chapter 14
Weight Loss from the Inside Out

Chapter 15
Nutrition for Mom and Baby

Chapter 16
Supplement/Product Recommendations

The Circle of Life – Nutritional Eating Guide

CHAPTER EIGHT

FATS & OILS – The Essential Balance

The fundamental understanding of fats and oils in the context of being good or bad is too simplified for what is a fairly complex relationship. What is possible is to take fats and oils apart, show you the pieces, and then explain how fats and oils are interrelated so that you will have the guidelines to choose your foods wisely.

Fats are the main form in which energy is stored in the body. A certain amount of fats are necessary in our diet. "Good" fats are important for the proper functioning of your entire body. Fats are crucial for lubricating our joints; are anti-inflammatory; are important for the immune system; balances our hormones (guys and gals); lend to hair, skin, and nail health, the digestive tract, neurological function, focus, brain power, and ultimately are crucial on the cellular level because every cell needs fats to function properly. Fats are critical for the bodies' nervous system. Of course, fats are important for insulation. The body would freeze to death without them. Women could not have babies without fat. So, as you can see, fats are critical for human life.

Fatty acids are the building blocks of fat. Essential fatty acids are external fats that our body does not produce, so we must consume them daily for the optimal balance of fat. So, what you must understand at this point is that a certain amount of fat is necessary in the diet because they provide our bodies with an adequate supply of essential fatty acids, and allow fat-soluble vitamins (vitamins A, D, E & K) to be efficiently absorbed in the intestines.

Fats are needed for their high-energy value. Triglycerides are one of the most plentiful fats in our body and in our food. When you eat fat and carbohydrates, they are generally broken down as triglycerides, and are either stored or transported throughout the body via the blood. Triglycerides are the chemical form of which fats exist in a food and our body, so therefore a triglyceride is the fundamental term for the essential fats found in all foods, which are classed as omega-3 and omega-6 fatty acids.

Essential Fatty Acids (EFA's)

The two acids classified as essential are omega-3 & omega-6. These two acids are not produced by the body, which makes them essential. They can only be supplied to the diet through foods, which includes oils. Omega-9 is also a fatty acid, but not essential because your body can produce it on its own. For example, the oil produced by the skin is the omega-9 produced by your body. The two main fatty acids, which make up the omega-9 family, are called stearic and oleic acid. Generally, omega-9 is also known as mono-unsaturated fat, most commonly found in Olive Oil.

Each class of fatty acid consists of a type of acid. The essential acids, omega-3 and 6, consist of acids found in foods. Omega-9 consists of acids produced both in the body and foods. It is important to understand that omega-3 and 6 are essential because they consist of acids that cannot be produced by the body, while omega-9, while present in many of the foods we eat, is unessential because your body can produce it on its own.

The chart below details each class of fatty acid, and the types assigned to each:

Classes and Sub-classes of Fatty Acids		
Omega-6	Omega-3	Omega-9
Essential Fatty Acid	Essential Fatty Acid	Non-Essential Fatty Acid
Polyunsaturated	Polyunsaturated	Monounsaturated
Linoleic Acid	Alpha linolenic acid	Oleic acid
GLA Gamma Linolenic acid	EPA	Stearic Acid
AA - Arachidonic Acid	DHA	
	Stearidonic Acid	

Omega-3 EFA's (polyunsaturated)

Experts agree that the typical western diet is deficient in omega-3 fatty acids because most people do not eat enough omega-3-rich foods. One of the most beneficial actions you can do to help prevent disease and other health problems is to increase your intake of the omega-3 fats. Omega-3 fats are high in two essential fatty acids, DHA and EPA. Omega-3 is found in fish, flaxseeds, chia seeds, macadamia nuts, walnuts, coconut oil, and dark green leafy vegetables, among many other foods. Please see the "Good Energy Food Sources of Omega 3 and 6" chart in this chapter for the full range of foods that are high in omega 3.

"Algal DHA is the healthiest form of **pure DHA and Omega 3** (fish get their DHA up the food chain from algae), and it does not endanger fish populations. It also does not contain any mercury or any other contaminant found in fish. The special algae are grown in environmentally sustainable tank farms, just as they grow spirulina. Several studies have shown that algal DHA is more easily utilized by the body. Also algal DHA does not have the saturated fat content that fish oil has, so algal DHA is actually better for the heart and arteries than fish (or krill) oil." This was C Admas' comment on Algal DHA who is a Naturopath who holds a Ph.D. in Natural Health Sciences, a Doctorate of Sciences in Integrative Health, and a degree in Traditional Naturopathy and more. (Refer to Chapter 16 for company recommendations for algal DHA).

Even those who eat fish twice a week are most likely not getting enough omega-3 EFA's. The optimal solution is to supplement with algal DHA, chia seeds, fish and/or flaxseed oil. EFA supplementation benefits not only general health, but can also be used therapeutically in higher dosages. EFA's have proven to aid in cardiovascular function, brain and nervous system functions, fat metabolism, skin health, joint flexibility, arthritis, ADD, and inflammation. Be sure to get the best quality fish oil, free of mercury, metals, PCBs, pesticides and dioxins. The oil should also be 3rd party tested, from deep-sea waters, such as the Arctic Ocean and Nordic Seas. The best processing procedure is "Molecular Distillation", which provides the purest quality and eliminates the undesirables. (Refer to Chapter 16 for product recommendations for Omega 3 EFA's).

Omega-6 EFA's (polyunsaturated)

Essential Fatty Acids are also classed as omega-6. Omega-6 EFA's are found in corn, soy, canola, safflower, sunflower, and many more foods.

Although necessary to your health, omega-6 fats should actually be minimized in our daily diets. Because the American diet consists of so much processed and refined foods, which are primarily made with omega-6 fats, our ratio of consumed essential fats is unhealthy and unbalanced. The ideal ratio of omega-6 to omega-3 fats is 1:1, however today the ratio favors omega-6 fats at averages ranging from 20:1 to 50:1. This imbalance can help cause a range of health problems.

While most people are consuming too many omega 6 fats, the majority are actually deficient in omega-6 Gamma-Linoleic Acid (GLA) because it is rarely found in foods. GLA has been used to assist in treating the following conditions: diabetes, eczema, osteoporosis, PMS, arthritis (due to its anti-inflammatory properties), skin ulcers, and breast disease. An excellent source of GLA is the supplement, Evening Primrose Oil (EPO), which comes from the seeds of the evening primrose plant. Other good supplements are Borage, Black Current Seed, and Hemp Seed oil.

Another essential fatty acid is Arachidonic acid. It is needed to help balance hormone groups that influence many of our bodily processes. When our bodies are in harmony and balance, every cell in the body functions properly. Some women who have cut fats out of their diet entirely either have irregular menstrual cycles and/or have gone through premature menopause.

When correcting their diet and using the proper type and amount of fats that are found naturally in whole foods, their menses returned to normal. Whole foods such as fish, vegetables, nuts, seeds, grains and legumes naturally contain the fats and oils our bodies require. The chart below lists food sources high in Omega 6 and 3 EFAs.

Omega-9 Fatty Acids (mono-unsaturated)

You might be getting the picture that because the omega-9 class of fatty acids is not deemed essential; that it is inherently of lesser importance. They are not essential because your body produces them by itself, but they do play an important part. Omega-9 is generally a mono-unsaturated fat found in many commonly consumed foods such as olive oil, avocado, almonds, peanuts, sesame oil, pecans, pistachio nuts, cashews, hazelnuts, macadamia nuts, and many others including fish oils to a small degree.

What is important to understand is that your body produces Omega-9 on its own so it does not need foods such as olive oil in high quantities. This becomes complicated because these same foods that have omega-9 fats also have varying levels of omega-3 and 6 fats. This is why foods must be examined individually according to its fatty acid make-up along with the many other factors that define their respective nutritional value.

Saturated vs. Unsaturated Fats

Oils are foods. Not all foods have fats, but all types of oils do have fats. Some oils are higher in essential fatty acids, Omega 3 and 6, while some are higher in non-essential fatty acids, Omega-9s. Most oils have combinations of all three classes. Foods (including oils) that have fat present have degrees of fatty acids and degrees of saturated and/or mono or poly-unsaturated fat molecules.

Saturated fats are solid at room temperature. For example, the fat on a steak is solid to the point where you can chew it. Likewise, butter is hard at room temperature. Saturated fat is found in all animal foods such as beef, pork, poultry, seafood, all dairy (milk, butter, cheese), and some vegetable oils (palm, palm kernel, coconut, cocoa butter, and hydrogenated oils).

Unsaturated fats are made up of the three classes of fatty acids explained above, omega 3, 6, and 9, which fall under the categories of poly or mono-unsaturated fats. The EFA chart on the previous page breaks down the different foods high in omega 3 and 6, which make them high in unsaturated fats.

To qualify saturated and unsaturated fats as good or bad would be shortsighted because many foods with fat contain levels of both. For example, butter fat is 60% saturated; 30% monounsaturated, and only 10% polyunsaturated. Sunflower seeds are 12% saturated; 21% monounsaturated and 67% polyunsaturated. Is butter less nutritious than sunflower oil? Before we can answer this and other related questions, we must understand both saturated and unsaturated fats in the context of their molecular structures, and how their chemical makeup defines the nutritional value of the fatty foods we eat.

Let's delineate saturated fats first. Simply put, there are saturated fats that are bad for your body known as long chain saturated fats (LCSF) and there are the good saturated fats, which are the short and medium chain saturated fats (MCSF & SCSF).

Long Chain Saturated Fats (LCSF)
These are the second most harmful fats next to hydrogenated oil, which we will learn about later in this section. "Long Chain" fats (I've dubbed them "longshanks") are the culprits behind unhealthy saturated fats. Longshanks are the reason saturated fats have such a bad reputation.

When longshanks are consumed, they are directed to the small intestine where bile salts must combine with the fats before the body can absorb them. This process creates toxic fat cells that peruse the veins and arteries creating storage and blockage. These have been proven to raise "bad" LDL blood cholesterol levels, contributing to heart disease. Longshanks are extremely concentrated. They carry many toxins, are difficult to break down, and are a key causal factor for obesity. They are found most commonly in animal products such as beef, pork, and chicken as well as dairy products, including milk and butter. Other sources of longshanks are palm oil and cottonseed oil -- both used extensively in processed foods. As we learned above, you can always recognize a saturated fat if it is solid at room temperature.

Medium Chain and Short Chain Saturated Fats (MCSF & SCSF)
Although our bodies do need a certain amount of saturated fats in our diet, they should come from "Medium and Short Chain" saturated fats, such as cold-pressed coconut oil. What makes these saturated fats "good" and actually vital to health is their ability to be absorbed directly by the liver, where they are

immediately available to the body and are sent out as a pure source of energy. These types of fatty acids are unlikely to cause obesity due to their quick digestion and energy conversion, never having the opportunity to be stored as body fat.

> ❖ **Coconut Oil**
> The coconut is highly nutritious and has fed and nourished people around the world for generations. It is classified as a "functional food" because of its numerous health benefits and nutritional content. Coconut oil is a combination of short and medium-chain saturated fats. Nearly 50% of the fatty acid in coconut oil is lauric acid. Lauric acid helps the body to fight against bacteria, yeast, fungi, and other viruses and immune disorders. Lauric acid also increases the metabolic rate, aiding in weight loss. *Remember, saturated fats are not aligned with any of the three classes of fatty acids, Omega 3, 6, and 9, because those fatty acids are all unsaturated fats. Lauric acid is only found within the MCSF's and SCSF's.*
>
> Coconut oil has long been used for its healing properties in traditional medicine among the Asian and Pacific populations. They consider it as a cure for all illness. Modern medicine has finally caught up to and confirmed the wide range of health benefits. Some such benefits include: anti-viral, anti-fungal, anti-bacterial; improves endurance, energy, digestion, bowel function, immune system function, cholesterol, free radical protection, thyroid function, loss of excess weight by increasing metabolic rate, the prevention of obesity and related problems, skin and hair health, and many more.
>
> Coconut oil is a stable type of cooking oil, with a smoking point above 400 degrees. Therefore, it is one of my favorites along with macadamia nut oil for cooking. Coconut oil tastes great in desserts, stir fry's, breads, melted on hot grains, on popcorn and used in the place of butter.

Unsaturated Fats (Mono and Poly)

Monounsaturated fats are not broken down by long or medium-short chains. These fats are most commonly found in some plants. You might remember that we defined omega-9 fatty acids as mono-unsaturated fats. Omega-9 fatty acids are produced by the body so they are not essential. This means that while foods with monounsaturated fats such as olive oil, cashews and avocados are great for the body in moderate amounts, they cause unnecessary fat storage when consumed in high quantities. Please understand that compressed oils extracted from the olive and macadamia nuts are liquid at room temperature, and thicken slightly when refrigerated (while saturated fats are solid at room temp.)

Polyunsaturated fats are also found in some plants, and usually in high concentrations. Like monounsaturated fats, whether refrigerated or left at room temperature, these fats remain in a liquid state. They are naturally found in sesame seeds, sunflower seeds, and most nuts. In their natural form, consumed as a whole food, these fats are good for you. When extracted and processed into most oils, they are no longer beneficial. Some of these highly refined oils are sunflower oil, safflower oil, soy oil and peanut oil. The three exceptions are Macadamia nut oil, Grapeseed oil, and Avocado oil.

Macadamia Nut Oil ("Mac Nut Oil") is over 80% unsaturated and contains no cholesterol. This oil is higher in polyunsaturated fats than any other source of fat, and contains a good amount of Vitamin E, a powerful anti-oxidant. Monosaturated fats have been shown to be the healthiest for the body and provide more antioxidants and health benefits than any other form of fat.

Mac Nut oil is more heat stable (410° smoke point) than Olive, Flax, Canola, Safflower or most other oils. Therefore, there is no danger of the harmful trans-fatty acids and free radicals forming as they can with other cooking oils. Its stability and versatility seems to make it the healthiest alternative to other cooking oils. It is a golden yellow color, has a buttery taste and tastes great in baked sweets or main dishes, dressings or stir-fry's.

Mac Nut Oil has the ideal ratio of omega-3 to omega-6 fatty acids (1:1). Where most processed foods and oils are so disproportionate with high amounts of omega-6's (contributing to arthritis, allergies and heart conditions), the Mac Nut oil can help lower the amount of omega-6 while increasing your Omega-3's.

Grapeseed Oil is the next best choice to Macadamia nut oil for cooking because its smoking point is 320 degrees. It is also very high in Vitamin E, linoleic acid, and contains more antioxidants than any other oil.

> ❖ **Hempseed Oil**
> This oil is a non-cooking oil, but it is a polyunsaturated fat relatively high (about 57%) in linoleic acid, or Omega 6. It is third highest to Borage and Primrose oil in the essential GLA. Although Hempseed oil is higher in Omega 6 than the popular Flaxseed oil (high in Omega 3), it is one of the best sources and very easily absorbed. It has one of the most ideal ratios of Omega 6 to Omega 3. It is true that Omega 6 & 3 fats, when heated and processed, are harmful, which is why most diets are lacking not only in Omega 3, but also a raw and natural source of Omega 6. The solution is taking raw, cold-pressed Hempseed oil regularly. I like to mix up my oils and take Flaxseed and Primrose oil one day and Hempseed oil the next. Like all aspects of nutrition, diversification is the key to finding balance.

The chart on the following page lists oils according to their fatty acid content.

Oils High in Omega 6, 3 and 9				
Oils	High in Omega 6	High in Omega 3	High in Omega 9	Saturated
Almond Oil	x		x	
Apricot Kernel Oil	x		x	
Avocado Oil	x		x	x
Black Currant Seed Oil	x		x	
Borage Oil	x		x	
Butter Fat	x			x
Canola Oil	x		x	
Coconut Oil	x		x	x (MCSF)
Cod Liver Oil	x		x	
Corn Oil	x			
Cotton Seed Oil	x	X		
Evening Primrose Oil		X		
Flaxseed Oil	x	x		
Grapeseed Oil	x			
Hazelnut Oil			x	
Hemp Seed Oil	x			
Lard	x			
Macadamia Nut Oil	x	X		
Olive Oil	x			
Palm Kernel Oil			x	x
Palm Oil	x			x
Peanut Oil	x		x	
Pistachio Oil			x	
Pumpkin Seed Oil	x		x	
safflower margarine	x		x	
Safflower Oil	x			
Salmon Oil		X		
Sardine Oil		X		
Sesame Seed Oil		X		
Soybean Oil	x			
Sunflower Seed Oil	x			
Vegetable Shortening	x			
Walnut Oil	x		x	
Wheat Germ Oil	x		x	

Fully Hydrogenated or Partially-Hydrogenated Oils

Hydrogenated oil is a saturated fat, and is the most dangerous fat you can ingest into your body. This is the one type of oil that could actually be considered worse than saturated fats. Whether vegetable oil is fully or partially hydrogenated makes no difference. Both manipulations are just as harmful. It is an unnatural oil imposter, usually extracted from soybean, cottonseed, palm, coconut, or other liquid oils. The oil begins as an unsaturated vegetable oil, extracted from plants, liquid at room temperature, and is then converted into solid, saturated shortening. The oil is then heated and processed to the point where its chemical structure has been altered to a Frankenstein like mutation. In simple terms, natural oil is being converted into a destructive synthetic substance. When oil is hydrogenated, its fatty acids are converted to the trans form, thus the term, Trans-fat. So, essentially, hydrogenated oil is a type of Trans-fatty acid. Trans-fatty acids can attach to your good cells in the body, mutate them, and over time possibly create disease and disorders. Trans-fat is the leading cause of bad cholesterol (LDL), which is the leading cause of heart disease, which is the leading killer of humans.

Hydrogenated oil is used for the mass production and preservation of highly refined or processed food. The reason these oils are made is for preservation. They increase the shelf life of food better than any other oil and many other preservatives. The process of producing hydrogenated oil is a result of the onset of the industrial revolution and evolution of mass production, which became standardized for most major industries in the 1930s, 40s, and 50s. The food industry was a natural fit for mass production because every person has to eat, and the practice of preserving food for the masses was thought of and still is perceived of as an awesome achievement. After all, saving a person from hunger is more important than feeding them nutritious food, right?

The fact is that mass production has little to do with helping people, and a lot to do with making profit from the hands and mouths of many. The bottom line for the processed food industry is that it is much cheaper to hydrogenate oil for the use of food production and preservation than to use naturally pressed oils that are more expensive, and do not preserve foods as long. The question for us as individuals is whether we can afford to cut so many corners with our health. That is what hydrogenated oil is produced for, cutting corners at the expense of you and your families' health. So be a strict gatekeeper when it comes to consuming processed foods and avoid hydrogenated oil at all costs.

How Fats & Oils Affect Cholesterol Levels

Now that we have defined the main types of fats, what should our relationship to them be? We have previously learned that fats are an essential part of life and that we must consume them on a daily basis. So how does fat consumption relate to cholesterol levels, and which omega fatty acids affect the good (HDL) and bad (LDL) cholesterol in the body? This is a crucial question and critical to understand because the processed food industry is not incentivized to educate you so most people consume high cholesterol foods for years, only realizing the truth after they are lying back in the hospital bed.

First let's make one thing clear and simple: cholesterol is only found in animals and their by-products. You won't find cholesterol in nuts, seeds, vegetables, and other plant foods. The body does make small amounts of cholesterol from saturated fats, in the liver. The body does need certain amounts of cholesterol, which is an important part of cell membranes and various other bodily functions.

What are the sources of good and bad cholesterol?

Trans-fatty acids (hydrogenated oils) are one of the main sources of bad cholesterol. As we have learned, hydrogenation is a harmful, chemical process that un-saturated oil goes through in order to become a hard, unnatural saturated fat. Trans-fats are found in these hydrogenated oils, along with animal sources including beef, pork, and lamb. Hydrogenated oil and trans-fats are also commonly found in commonly consumed highly processed foods including margarine, crackers, cookies, doughnuts, French fries, and white bread. These chemical-laden, dangerous fats are identified as some of the most dangerous and harmful groups of fat. Not only have they been linked to increasing LDL levels, they also appear to lower the good cholesterol (HDL). This is especially true when hydrogenated oil and trans-fats replace a majority of the natural dietary oils, such as Omega 3, 6, and 9.

Saturated fats are also a primary source of bad cholesterol. Long chain saturated fats (the harmful "Longshanks") are mainly found in animal and dairy products. It does not take a nutritionist to realize why heart disease is the number one killer of Americans since animal and dairy products most likely make up over half of the average American's food intake.

The good news is that we can take advantage of our diet to correct this imbalance of cholesterol. Polyunsaturated and monounsaturated fats (Omega 3, 6 and 9), mostly found in plants, and are not linked to increasing LDL. In fact, they have actually been proven to help decrease LDL and even increase HDL. Also, if your diet consists of mostly poly and mono-unsaturated fats, only small amounts of animal cholesterol and saturated fats, and no hydrogenated oils, than your HDL/LDL balance should continue to improve, effectively lowering your LDL and keeping your HDL at the proper level.

Oil in Moderation

Why does food need oil? Why was oil ever used in the first place? What is the purpose? Oil was developed and used in food preparation for flavor, as a lubricant, for preservation, and for consistency. All oils are processed in one way or another. There is no natural occurring oil, except through some form of extraction. Flaxseeds don't simply "bleed" out their oil content. The oil must be pressed out and extracted. What I want to convey is that oils, no matter how nutritious, should be consumed in moderation.

Did you know that it takes about 40 ears of corn to make only a few ounces of corn oil? That proves how concentrated even 1 Tbsp of oil is and why it is not as easily absorbed as eating an ear of corn, which has only a fraction of oil in comparison. If you are going to eat oil or take flaxseed oil, primrose oil, hempseed oil, fish oil, or any others, make sure it is raw, cold-pressed, and organic. Fish oil supplements should be molecularly distilled and free of all mercury, PCB's and metals. Cold-pressed means the oil has not been cooked, so the enzymes and nutrients have not been killed. If you cook or heat oil, you will also destroy its nutrients. The only oils I cook with, which have high smoking points, are coconut, grape seed, macadamia nut, and avocado oil. All other oils are best used in their raw, cold-pressed state, such as olive oil.

Fats and oils can be healing or harmful. Use what I have presented in this chapter to make wise choices about which foods and oils you consume. Energy is directly affected by the good and bad fats. I encourage you to eat and cook with the fats and oils I have recommended. Moderation is the key. On your path towards just good energy, minimizing and eliminating the harmful fats (hydrogenated, saturated, cholesterol), while replacing them with healthful fats (Omega 3, 6 and 9), will change your life.

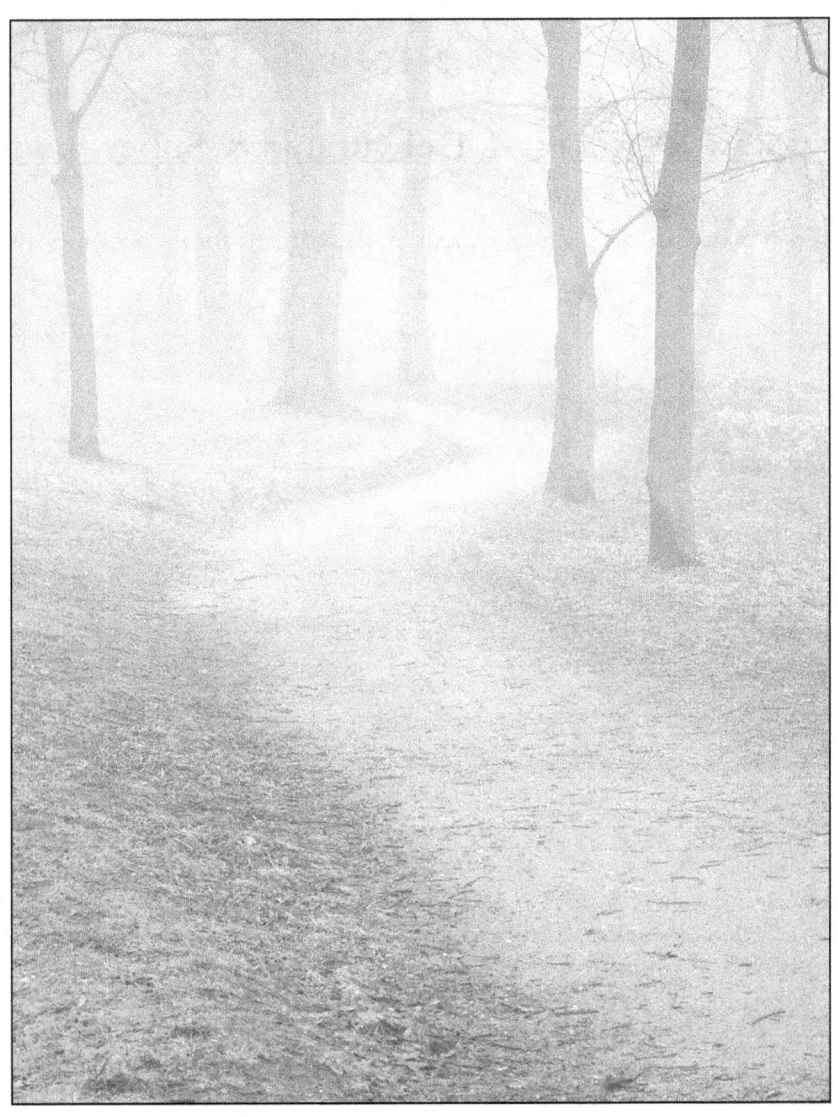

"It's bizarre that the produce manager is more important to my children's health than the pediatrician." ~ Meryl Streep

CHAPTER NINE

Raw, Fermented, Dehydrated & Super-foods

Non-cooked foods can be classified as raw, fermented, dehydrated foods, and super-foods which include:

- ❖ Grains
- ❖ Flours
- ❖ Fermented or cultured foods
- ❖ Tofu
- ❖ Tempeh
- ❖ Nuts and seeds
- ❖ Dehydrated foods
- ❖ Fruits and vegetable
- ❖ Green Super-foods
- ❖ Red Super-foods

Let's explore each of these classes:

Grains

Whenever people talk about grains, they tend to think about bread. For centuries bread has been a food staple of most cultures. Our ancestors usually soaked their grains and dried them in the sun before making bread, which often left the center of the bread raw, which made the bread easier to digest. Today, most bread is made from bleached white or wheat flour with added chemicals. Bread is so over-cooked now that it has little or no nutritional value and definitely no life-giving enzymes. Whole wheat, whole grain and sourdough breads made from whole grains are better, but they still lack enzymes to aid digestion. For bread to be nutritious, it should be made from sprouted dried grains and, when possible, baked by the sun or in a dehydrator.

Grains come from grass seeds and they are essential to our body. Whether you eat your grains raw or cooked, all grains should ideally be soaked and sprouted. That way you can receive all of the minerals, vitamins and protein available in that grain.

Whole grains contain amylase, a digestive enzyme that helps to break the grain down. Even if the whole grain is cooked, like brown rice, the enzyme retains some potency.

What is Gluten?
Grain (especially wheat) protein is what makes up gluten. It is a protein-carbohydrate mixture that is mainly contained in wheat, oats, barley, rye and spelt. Some people have sensitivity to gluten that is usually either intestinal (gastro-intestinal tract is the most affected organ) or allergy-related (allergies develop due to the

proteins in the gluten). Even those without gluten intolerance generally have some difficulty digesting too much gluten at any given time. Gluten is difficult on the digestive tract and can irritate the bowel. The most commonly developed disease due to the forming of gluten-allergies is Celiac disease. Celiac disease is partly due to the inability to break down gluten (malabsorption). I strongly recommend minimizing the amount of glutinous flour you consume. It is best to eat glutinous grains sprouted first and then cooked or ground into flour. Now let's explore glutinous grains versus non-glutinous grains:

Glutinous grains: Barley, Oats, Rye, and Wheat

Barley - There are two kinds; Scotch barley, which is a whole grain, and pearl barley, which is refined. Soak barley for one day only, or it may sour. Do not sprout it.

Oat Groats - Oat groats are difficult to find truly raw. Because insects prey so severely on raw oats, many growers choose to lightly steam the oats prior to shipping to kill the insects. The groats can be soaked but will not sprout unless you find the "sprouting variety" that has not been steamed.

Rolled Oats - These are oats that have been processed. If you choose to eat oats, soak them for 10-15 minutes in warm water. They are great at breakfast topped with a sweet sauce. Because of their sticky consistency, they can also be ground up in burgers, vegetable nut loaves or sauces.

Rye - Rye has a sour flavor and is great for making breads and crackers. Try adding caraway or dill to recipes that call for rye.

Spelt - (Kamut) This is a non-hybrid wheat that originated in Egypt. People who have difficulty digesting wheat, due to the gluten, should have little difficulty digesting foods made with spelt. Although spelt has some gluten, it is less than the quantity in wheat. It soaks and sprouts like wheat berries.

Wheat Berries - When soaked and sprouted, this grain is soft and chewy. It can be ground up and made into crackers, cookies or dehydrated breads. Wheat berries can be sprouted, planted into soil and grown into wheat grass. Wheat is the highest grain in gluten, which is why many have difficulty digesting this grain and commonly have allergies to it. However, once the grain is soaked and sprouted it is much easier to digest.

Non-glutinous grains: Amaranth Rice, Buckwheat, Corn, Millet, Quinoa, Non-white Rice

Amaranth - This is an Inca grain, low in gluten. It can be used as a replacement for wheat in breads and crackers.

Buckwheat Groats - This is a strong-flavored grain that is high in protein, B Vitamins, and calcium. It is easily digested and very gentle on the stomach.

Corn - Popcorn kernels and whole dried corn are very difficult to soften. Corn does not sprout. It is a starchy grain and more difficult to digest than most other grains, except for wheat.

Millet - Millet is high in protein, potassium, calcium, iron, and vitamin B. It has a bland flavor, but it is very satisfying.

> ❖ **Quinoa** - This grain originated in South America and is now grown in Colorado. Quinoa is a complete protein, has ten times more absorbable iron than wheat and corn and is high in Vitamin B. It is gluten-free and one of the least starchy grains. It is very easily digested and is one of my favorites to both eat raw and

Rice - I recommend six basic varieties of rice: long grain brown rice, short grain brown rice, brown jasmine rice, and short grain sweet brown rice, wild rice and Basmati rice. I use only the brown variety, as the white is highly refined. Short grain brown and short grain sweet brown rice both have a stickier texture and are great to use for sushi or in grain burgers and nut loaves. Basmati rice, which originated in India, has a nutty flavor. Wild rice is a long, dark grain with a strong distinct flavor. We like to mix it with other varieties of rice.

> ❖ **Tip on Sprouting Rice -** When sprouting rice, allow it to grow only very short tails, otherwise the flavor becomes very strong.

Tapioca - Tapioca is made from the root of the Cassava plant. The most widely available forms are tapioca flour (also called cassava flour) and pearl tapioca. The flour is used as a thickening agent for soups, fruit fillings, glazes, gravies, etc. Tapioca flour can replace corn starch in recipes, and also can be used as a good alternative to other thickening agents. Tapioca has become more widely used recently because it is a gluten-free starch. The small, starchy pearl tapioca granules are used to make tapioca pudding and to thicken pie fillings. Because foods made from whole grain flours tend to be heavier and dense, we found that substituting approximately ¼ the amount of the grain flour with tapioca flour, helped them to be lighter and easier to digest.

Flours

Many of the grains we have spoken of can be ground into flours in their raw state but are more nutritious when soaked, sprouted, dried and then ground into flours.

An interesting note on flour: In the 1930s and 1940s the Food and Drug Administration (FDA) prohibited highly refined white flour from crossing state lines because, at that time, it was considered a poison. Today not only is it shipped across state lines; it is shipped to many parts of the world. Regulations and standards have definitely changed!

Just because the government now says refined flour is okay does not mean we should include it in our diets. Refined flours are milled until the fiber and nutrients are removed, then some chemicals are added back in to replace those vitamins and minerals which have been stripped! These flours are found in many of the processed foods consumed in a typical American diet. It takes our bodies up to 72 hours to digest refined flours because of the loss of fiber. In our digestive tract, these flours are like a paste -- clogging up our colons, poisoning our system and interfering with normal digestion.

Nuts and Seeds

Nuts and seeds are an excellent source of protein and calcium and are very important to a healthy lifestyle. They are rich in Vitamin B, B-Complex vitamins, copper, phosphorous, calcium, iron, magnesium, and potassium. They contain unsaturated fat, which means they are easy to digest--with seeds being easier to digest than nuts. Either can be eaten right out of the shell, soaked in filtered water, or sprouted. Their nutritional value is enhanced and they become less fatty if they are soaked.

Soaked nuts and seeds can be used to make nut milks, seed cheese and seed yogurt, sauces, patés, dressings, and desserts. Soaked almonds, cashews, and sesame seeds are best if kept in airtight glass jars in the refrigerator. They should be rinsed every couple of days to maintain freshness.

After soaking, all nuts and seeds can be dehydrated by placing them on a dehydrator tray and dehydrating at 115 degrees for about 14-16 hours. This will increase their time of freshness. Once soaked and dehydrated, these raw nuts and seeds can be stored in a refrigerator or freezer to prevent rancidity and oxidation. However, if raw nuts and seeds are used within two weeks, they can be stored in an airtight container in the pantry.

Raw nuts and seeds contain enzyme inhibitors, making them very difficult to digest and break down. Fortunately these inhibitors are released by soaking in water for a minimum of 8-12 hours. This process increases the nutrient content of the nut or seed, eliminates almost half of the fat, increases the enzyme content and creates a highly alkaline food. A soaked nut and seed becomes easily digestible and the fat, vitamins and minerals are easily assimilated. See Chapter 2 for more details on the importance of soaking and sprouting.

Let's learn about the different types of edible nuts:

Cashews - Cashews are not truly raw because they must be slightly steamed to harvest them. They are very dirty nuts, so make sure to wash them with a vegetable cleanser. Cashews are very soft and can absorb chemicals easily, but they can also throw them off easily. The oils from cashews float easily to the surface when soaked. They are high in Pantothenic Acid or Vitamin B-5, an important B Vitamin that is useful in reducing stress and anxiety.

Pecans – A good source of omega fatty acids and should be soaked to decrease the acidity.

Macadamia Nuts - A hard nut. They are sweet like cashews but more expensive. They are very high in monounsaturated fats, Omega-3 fatty acids, and Vitamin E. They also have a resistance to high temperatures, making the oil ideal for cooking with.

> ❖ **Almonds** - Almonds are grown in much the same way as fruits. In their early growth stages, they resemble large pitted fruits like plums, nectarines, apricots, and peaches. Almonds grow in a tough greenish hull that looks like a peach hull. When the almond ripens, the hull splits open and produces the almond in its inner shell. Almonds contain all eight of the essential amino acids – that means they are a complete protein! Almonds are available year round and can be stored easily. They are a good source of Omega Fatty Acids and one of the most alkaline foods, so eat or drink up!
>
> ❖ **Walnuts** - Clean them with fruit and vegetable wash before soaking. Although walnuts are known for being acidic, soaking them decreases the acidity. They are high in Omega 3 Fatty Acids, Vitamin E and are a good source of monounsaturated fats.

Pine Nuts - These nuts have an unusually strong pine flavor that is great for pesto.
Now, let's learn about the different types of edible seeds.

Pumpkin Seeds - (Pepitas) They are green, flat seeds with a distinctive flavor that is enhanced by soaking. The oil of the seed is commonly used by men with prostate problems and is good for general urinary tract health.

Sesame Seeds - Small round seeds. They can be ground and made into a "butter", called tahini, which has a rich cream flavor. Tahini is very high in calcium.

Sunflower Seeds - High in vitamins A and D and rich in protein. They can be soaked or sprouted in their raw state. They can also be planted and grown into sunflower greens, also known as sunflower sprouts. These are great tasting when soaked and sprouted into tall greens. Sunflower greens taste great on salads and sandwiches and are high in chlorophyll, protein, minerals and energy. They have a nutty flavor and are fairly easy to sprout, see sprouting procedures in Chapter 20.

Chia Seeds - These tiny nutritious seeds were a staple for the Aztecs and Native American Indians. Chia seeds were their power foods that gave them strength, endurance and sustained them nutritionally on long journeys. Chia seeds are rich in protein (about 7g per serving), omega fatty acids, fiber, provides 35% calcium (5x more calcium than milk per serving) and 30% iron per serving! They provide long lasting energy fuel and supply of electrolytes, keeping the body hydrated for long periods of time. It seems that nature created a food that can nourish, hydrate and energize the body specifically for long durations – the ideal athlete food!

They are also the ideal workaholic food – sustained energy and nutrition without having to eat large quantities of food. I would go further to say it is ideal for toddlers who are too busy playing to stop and eat along with pregnancy, the time when your body needs the best absorbable nutrients and hydration.

When you soak chia seeds in water they create a gel-like texture which when eaten slows down the conversion of carbohydrates into sugar, making them ideal for diabetics. This slow conversion process creates sustained energy and keeps the body from energy crashing.

The bonus is that soaked chia seeds help to lean out the waistline due to their ability to control carbohydrate absorption (you won't store the carbs as fat); their ability to cleanse the colon; nourish the body, keeping it satisfied and less hungry (craving less sweets); clean out bad fats; give you more energy to exercise.

❖ **Flax Seeds -** When soaked they have a gelatin-like consistency, which can be great for thickening sauces and dressings. Soaked and well-rinsed flaxseeds can be dried and ground into meal. They are the best whole food source of the essential fatty acid called linolenic, otherwise known as Omega 3. Of all the nuts and seeds, flax seeds contribute most to optimum cellular function, eliminating the storage of bad fats in the body and helping in the regeneration of your body. They are good for joint health and for raising HDL (good cholesterol) levels. Flaxseed meal and oil are available in the supplement form. Most people should take 1000 to 1500 mg. of flax oil daily. It is a good alternative for fish oil, especially for those with diabetes who cannot take fish oil.

Flaxseeds are not absorbable unless they have been ground up first. Once ground, they are referred to as flaxseed meal. <u>Flaxseed meal</u> is a great addition to the diet because it is a gentle fiber, filled with nutrients, amino acids, vitamins and omega fatty acids. Flaxseed meal is a great fiber source because it glides gently through the digestive tract, due to its fat content, pulling out toxins along the way. One to two tablespoons daily is generally recommended.

❖ **Hempseeds** – Chinese Records dating back to 16th century B.C, document hemp as one of their primary and most consistent crops. Hemp has also been an important nutrient to many other cultures throughout history, such as the Egyptians and Aztecs. Hemp seed is a little over one third protein, about one half fat, and just over ten percent carbohydrates (mostly from the fiber). Hempseeds are an excellent source of Essential Fatty Acids, particularly in linoleic Acid, or Omega 6, and GLA. Hempseeds also provide an excellent complete protein source, and are balanced in all of the essential Amino Acids. Hempseed protein powder is the most natural and easily digested protein powder available, far superior to soy protein. See the pros and cons of Soy in Chapter 10. Hemp is available in the forms of oil, seed butter, hulled seeds, and protein powder (ground up hempseeds). (See chapter 8 for more information on hempseed oil.)

Fermented or Cultured Foods

Our stomach and bowels need an acidic state for easy digestion. I know that sounds contrary to the whole idea of reaching a more alkaline state in our bodies, but we must have a balance of acid to alkaline in our system. As with everything in nature, especially within our bodies, there must always be a balance for things to function properly. For example, we can't breathe in oxygen all day, we need that balance of breathing out carbon dioxide; we can't stay awake all day, our bodies must have a balance of sleep; we can't eat only fats and protein, we must eat carbohydrates also. Same goes with the balance of acid to alkaline in our body. The acidic measurement, PH, of the stomach can go as low as 1.0 to 3.0 (extremely acidic), while the blood strives to be around 7.0 to 7.4 (more neutral). The stomach must have a high acidity to help break down bacteria from foods and secrete digestive juices such as bile and pepsin in order to break down proteins. See Chapter 13 for more reasons why the balance between acid and alkaline is essential.

To help restore and maintain the necessary acidity in our digestive tract, our diet should include some fermented or cultured foods. The first step to fermenting or culturing grains, nuts, seeds and legumes is soaking them in water to break down the digestive inhibitors and increase the nutrient content. The next step is fermentation or culturing, which actually increases the enzyme content. Fermentation and culturing is the process of breaking a food down through enzymes, probiotics, heat, etc, over a period of time.

Kombucha Tea, detailed in Chapter 13 is fermented naturally by letting the tea sit at room temperature for 3-4 weeks. Yogurt is cultured and fermented by taking the milk, adding probiotics (acidophilus cultures) and letting it sit for an extended period of time. The enzymes, probiotics and nutrients increase rapidly and actually pre-digest themselves. All that means is that the enzymes created during the fermentation and culturing, actually break down the food, creating little to no digestive effort once consumed into our bodies. Because predigested foods require less digestive work and no extra enzyme output from your own enzyme pool, your body can assimilate the vital nutrients these foods contain.

Examples of fermented and cultured foods and beverages are:

- ❖ Nut yogurts
- ❖ Seed cheeses
- ❖ Yogurt
- ❖ Coconut Kefir
- ❖ Coconut Aminos (raw organic coconut-based condiment to use in place of soy sauce)
- ❖ Kombucha Tea
- ❖ Nama Shoyu (natural, raw soy sauce)
- ❖ Probiotics (acidophilus, bifidus, FOS)
- ❖ Miso (fermented soybean or garbanzo paste, commonly found in Miso Soup)
- ❖ Sourdough
- ❖ Sprouted raw breads
- ❖ Raw sauerkraut
- ❖ Raw pickles
- ❖ Raw pickled vegetables
- ❖ Fermented grain drinks

How to Ferment for Food and Beverage Creation

Fermenting nuts, grains, seeds and legumes is actually very easy:

❖ After soaking and/or minimal sprouting, blend them in a blender
❖ Add water and pour into a glass jar.
❖ Cover the top with a loose fitting lid and leave the jar out on a counter for 6 to 24 hours, depending on the recipe.

> ❖ Fermented grain drinks take longer to ferment -- about two to three days. Adding already fermented foods such as miso, or replacing the water with a fermented grain drink adds more friendly bacteria and plant enzymes.

When eaten daily, these fermented or cultured foods change the colon from an unhealthy alkaline state to a healthy acidic one. The fats, starches, and proteins in whole foods that have been fermented have been broken down into more simple compounds, and therefore digest more easily.

What is Tofu?

Tofu is made from soybeans, water and a natural coagulant. It is sold in cakes or blocks packed in water. It is processed much like cheese and is a good meat and dairy substitute. It has no cholesterol. Most of the fat in tofu is polyunsaturated and contains lecithin, a substance which is believed to help dissolve fat in the body. However, it is not the easiest protein source to digest and can tax your organs when over-consumed. Tofu is not a necessary part of the diet.

If you choose to use tofu, make sure it is organic and ideally sprouted. Tofu is a cooked food, so for those who are pursuing a more live diet, sprouted nuts, seeds, and grains are a better source of easily digested protein and calcium.

Eat in moderation: Although tofu and other soybean products have been raved about for their protein, nutrients, and cancer-fighting abilities, this does not mean you should over-eat these foods on a daily basis. Limit your intake of processed soy in any form and try to avoid processed soy products including soy milk, cheese, fake soy-based meats and soy protein powder.

> ❖ **What is Tempeh?** Tempeh, like tofu, is also made from soybeans. However, the main difference between these two soy based foods is tempeh's higher protein and nutrient content and easier to digest quality. Tempeh is created from cultured and fermented soybeans. In one block of tempeh, there is about 50-60 grams of protein and a very high amount of calcium and other minerals. You get the most nutrients from tempeh if it is eaten raw, because any heating will kill some of the nutrients. Crumble it on salad; add it to stir fry after cooking, or eat it raw dipped in a teriyaki sauce. It is a great part of a meal or snack that gives you energy and satisfaction. Tempeh is considered a pre-digested food due to its high content of enzymes so where some people get bloated after eating tofu or plain soybeans, tempeh is very easy to assimilate and digest in the body.

Dehydrated Foods

The dehydration process has been around for centuries; our ancestors used the sun or fire to dry their food surplus. In Egypt, dried foods have been found in pyramids, entombed for centuries with their nutritional value intact!

Dehydration is a simple, healthy and delicious way of preserving live foods. By regulating the flow of heat and air, the dehydrator evaporates the water content of the food. Microorganisms cannot grow without moisture; therefore dehydrated foods can be preserved for a long time. Due to the shrinkage that occurs during drying, dehydrated food takes up much less storage space, and they no longer need to be refrigerated. It is great survival food.

Dehydration removes the water, leaving the essential vitamins, proteins, minerals, fats, carbohydrates, and plant enzymes largely intact. Dehydrated food loses only 25 percent of its nutritional value. By contrast, Live Foods lose their enzymes and therefore their nutritional value, when heated over 115 degrees. Other processing methods, such as canning, baking and boiling, require temperatures of 212 degrees or higher. Temperatures can vary in dehydrators. Dehydrate at less than 110 degrees to ensure the food's nutritional value.

Super-foods

If foods could wear a cape and fly around saving people, they would be the foods that are classified as 'Super-foods'. These foods are heroic in the sense that they are designed exclusively for the purpose of improving and maintaining a healthy balance of body and mind. There is nothing not to like about super-foods and whether red or green, I highly recommend them. Let's explore:

Green Super-foods

Green grasses, also known as <u>Cereal Grass</u>, have been around for thousands of years. Cereal grass is the young green plant which grows to produce the cereal grain (wheat, barley, oat, rye, etc.) The young grasses are very different and far superior nutritionally from the mature seed or grain. The nutrient profile is slightly higher in cereal grasses compared to dark green leafy vegetables. Ancient Oriental and Middle Eastern cultures consumed the young grass plants of wheat and barley. In the 1930's, Cereal Grass, was the main supplement promoted for nutrient deficiencies and other illnesses. Prior to the development of synthetic vitamin supplements, dried grass tablets were actually recommended by doctors and known by scientists and the general public to be healing and essential to the diet.

Unfortunately, with the discovery of isolating and creating individual vitamins and minerals and the growth of the pharmaceutical industry, the precious cereal grasses were forgotten. If you think about nature, there is no such thing as 1500 mg of calcium in a single chunk, or even a single isolation of vitamin C. Although taking low doses of multi vitamins and minerals can help fill in the gap of a lacking diet, why not get those very nutrients in a whole absorbable food that your body recognizes? Why not consume these amazing super-foods daily and reap the full benefits?

In the 1960's and 70's some doctors and scientists began revisiting the use of cereal grasses. Dr. Ann Wigmore began growing and chewing young blades of wheat grass and soon recovered from her illness that had been medically "untreatable". She continued to extend her research and therapeutic use on patients with many ailments, having much success. Also, Dr Yoshihide Hagiwara began studying the dietary benefits of cereal grasses. He too was able to improve his degenerative health through the cereal grasses. Dr. Hagiwara found that "the leaves of the cereal grasses provide the nearest thing to the perfect food that this planet offers", and stated, "I have come to believe that the true medicine is young green barley and wheat leaves which are eaten by human beings as staple food….Such grasses are as indispensable as the elements are".

Many cereal grass producers will juice the freshly cut grasses. This is fine if you are going to consume the juiced grass immediately. However, once the grass is juiced, it oxidizes quickly, resulting in valuable nutrient loss. Furthermore, many producers wet mill or spray this juice into a powder. A carrier such as maltodextrin is typically used in order to enhance the flavor and make the juice powder more water soluble. Maltodextrin adds empty calorie carbohydrates and has a glycemic index similar to sugar. A properly grown, processed and stored whole-leaf cereal grass powder offers up to 25 times more nutrition per serving and is considered a whole food, green leafy vegetable that your body can absorb and assimilate nutrients much better.

A green super-food blend includes many varieties of raw greens -- especially the grasses, sea vegetables, blue-green algae and chlorophyll. These important foods are rarely consumed in the diet and provide more nutrients combined than a typical multi-vitamin, as discussed previously. Taking a combination of greens provides a full spectrum of vitamins, minerals, antioxidants, amino acids, omegas, enzymes, fibers and proteins. These whole foods are excellent for the immune system and digestive system, for mental health, cholesterol control, and the proper balance and functioning of all of the body's organs and systems.

You need plenty of raw greens and sprouts. Most people do not eat or drink enough greens. We find that if we use a super-food green mixture in addition to our green drinks and salads, we get enough greens, and guess what? The good and sustained energy boost is fantastic!

> ❖ After years of researching and sampling several green super-food products, my family prefers <u>Vitamineral Green's</u>, <u>Amazing Grass's Green Super-food</u>, <u>Catie's Greens</u>, <u>Dr. Tony's Vibrant Greens</u>, and <u>Green Magma Plus</u>. See product recommendations in Chapter 16. The ingredients in all of these products are of the absolute highest quality, which include varieties of green grasses, chlorophyll, blue-green and sea algae, probiotic cultures (lactobacilli and acidophilus), natural raw fibers, antioxidants, and omega fatty acids.

Red Super-foods: Health-Promoting Berries/Fruits

There are various fruits and berries, which are vital to health, especially in this day and age of environmental pollutants and daily stresses. The most researched and important Red fruits, which I have included as daily recommendations are as follows:

- ❖ **Gogi Berries (Wolf Berries)**
- ❖ **Schizandra Berries**
- ❖ **Pomegranates**
- ❖ **Acai Fruit**
- ❖ **Rhodiola Berry**
- ❖ **Grapes/Grapeseed**
- ❖ **Lycopene (extract from Tomatoes)**
- ❖ **Mangosteen Plant**
- ❖ **Red and Purple Berries such as Blueberries**
- ❖ **Cranberries**
- ❖ **Bilberries**

All of the fruits above should be categorized as "Powerful Antioxidant Super-foods".

You should be aware that the average American ingests at least 300 lbs. of chemicals/pollutants/pesticides per year. Think about all of the chemicals and preservatives in our foods and the toxic gases and carcinogenic chemicals parading through the atmosphere. It is a tribute to the durability of the human body that the rates of cancer and other diseases aren't even higher.

Eating a healthy and organic diet is only part of the solution. Every person should be supplementing with Antioxidant-Rich super-foods. They have been proven by health professionals and scientists to fight and deactivate the hundreds of pollutants and pesticides we inhale and ingest daily. You might have seen food labels with an "O.R.A.C" number, or a claim that the food is "high on the ORAC scale". The breakdown of O.R.A.C. is "Oxygen Radical Absorbency Capacity". This scale was developed as a method of measuring antioxidant contents in different foods such as berries, fruits, vegetables, cacao, wine, etc. All it simply means is that certain foods contain higher amounts of antioxidants which can absorb and "fight" free radicals and pollutants in the body.

The following health-promoting characteristics are shared by these powerful fruits:
High in antioxidants, minerals, amino acids, trace minerals, energy, stamina, and are anti-inflammatory, alkalizing, boosts the immune system, powerhouse of nutrition, anti-aging, environmental protectors, stimulates mental function, and balances the nervous system.

I recommend taking a combination of the fruits daily in a concentrated/fresh powder or juice. There are various companies that have developed amazing combinations of powder versions of all or most of these fruits combined.

> ❖ Catie's Vitamin C powder and Dr. Tony's "Pomegranate Power" are two products which are high on the ORAC scale, about 5,000, and are loaded with all of the berries and other high antioxidant fruits. They taste great and have become part of my daily regime. I mix the dried fruit powder in water and drink first thing in the morning on an empty stomach. See Chapter 16 for more information on these products.

Superfood Sweetener: Yacon Syrup

Yacon syrup is the latest sweetener from Peru. It is considered by many as a nutritious superfood that is low in sugars and rich in vitamins and minerals.

"Straight from the rich, fertile soil of Peru, *Yacon* Root is the latest unique, superfood finding its way to the consumer market as the most healthy, nutritious sweetener! *Yacon* is rich in Potassium, Phosphorus, Chromium, Calcium, Iron, Copper, and other trace minerals. It contains a whole B complex profile, important antioxidants and 11% complete protein by dry weight. Use it as you would any sweetener -- in food recipes and in beverages, teas, coffee, smoothies, etc."
(Darin Olien, Darin's Naturals) www.darinsnaturals.com

CHAPTER
TEN

Processed Foods

The processing and refining of food is unfortunately a very common practice. A processed food is any food that has been altered from its natural state by any method, such as refining. Refining is simply a form of processing, where food has been altered and generally stripped of its original raw fiber, fats and/or nutrients. Processed and refined foods and oils have a longer shelf-life, but provide absolutely no health benefits. The most commonly refined foods include grains (white flour, white rice), sugars (white sugar), salt (refined salt) and oils (refined vegetable oils). These processed and refined foods that have been transformed from a whole food to a synthetic food are quickly absorbed into the bloodstream, creating high glucose levels and acid, which usually ends up as stored fat. These processed and refined foods and oils are one of the leading causes of today's rise in degenerate diseases and frequent illnesses. See chapter 13 for more information on how processed foods and acid can ravage a body.

After decades of consuming the most highly refined food products, people are beginning to realize that we actually need ALL of what food provides, not just the fragmented remains. The processing & refining process removes most of the fiber and vitamins, which are needed for our body to properly digest the food and maintain optimal health. The fiber that has been removed from foods that are processed is necessary to help transport the nutrients and food itself to the designated areas in the body. Eating foods without fiber is like a bicycle manufacturer creating a bike without tires, and expecting it to get you where you want to go. It is absurd.

The industrialized diet today is a trend towards mass production and factory processing, containing large proportions of refined foods, very opposite from the natural foods diet that was so prominent before the 20th century. Refined white flour and white sugar are the two basic components. These "new" foods often have additives and preservatives to allow for packaging, shipping, and "shelf life".

With the introduction and use of refined foods we have seen a significant rise in heart disease, diabetes, cancer and tooth decay.

The FDA continues to ignore the health-injuring effects of processed foods. Instead, they promote the following reasons for processing and refining: to improve shelf life or storage time; to increase the nutritional value *(The flaw here is that they add synthetic vitamins to foods because many important vitamins and minerals are processed out of the whole food)*; to make food more available; to improve the flavor of foods; to make foods easier to prepare; and to improve consumer acceptance *(color & appearance)*.

Unfortunately, the refined and fast food diet has become one of the greatest economic supporters of our currently expensive medical system. The diseases generated by this industrial diet have created great wealth for pharmaceutical and medical professionals.

Let's drill down in to the various types of processed foods:

- ❖ Pastas
- ❖ Sugars
- ❖ Artificial Sweeteners
- ❖ Additives
- ❖ Irradiated Foods
- ❖ Table Salt
- ❖ Genetically Modified Foods
- ❖ Processed Soy Products

Pasta

Many types of pasta have dairy, refined oils, such as refined olive oil and canola oil, eggs and preservatives in their ingredients, so read the labels carefully. Try vegetable pastas made without eggs, and made only from whole grain flours. Wheat pastas are the most common variety, but quinoa, spelt, corn, rice, and amaranth pastas are easier to digest. Also consider Asian varieties such as Udon, a broad type of Japanese pasta made from brown rice and/or wheat, and Soba, a thin Japanese pasta usually made from wheat and buckwheat with ingredients such as mugwort and mountain yam. Asian pastas are usually nutritionally superior to American refined pastas.

Most pasta is made with refined white flour – avoid at all costs. The more refined the grain, the longer it sits in the digestive tract. It often takes 72 hours for pasta to digest, and your body will absorb little to no nutritional value. Instead, the refined flour is making your system work harder, creating negative energy value. An alternative is to make your own pasta, using organic, whole grain flour.

Sugar

Refined white sugar, also one of the worst *simple carbohydrates*, is a "complete chemical" that has been extracted from plants. It contains no protein, no fiber, no fat, no vitamins or useful minerals. It has no enzymes or trace elements. In other words, it has no food value whatsoever. It has been linked to heart disease, obesity, kidney failure, diabetes, blindness, and tooth decay.

An excess of processed sugars in the diet could lead to symptoms such as:
- ❖ Heart disease
- ❖ Excess weight
- ❖ Fatigue and frequent sleepiness
- ❖ Depression
- ❖ Lack of mental clarity
- ❖ Kidney failure
- ❖ Blindness
- ❖ Tooth decay
- ❖ Bloating

❖ Low blood sugar
❖ High blood pressure
❖ High triglycerides

False Energy

Sugar is promoted as a source of quick energy, but it has failed in that category, too. Although it is a simple carbohydrate, it ultimately causes a loss of energy. During the refining process, sugar is completely stripped of fiber that would otherwise help slow down its absorption into the system. When it is eaten in any quantity, the bloodstream is rapidly overloaded with glucose, creating that sugar "high". Large amounts of insulin have to be released from the pancreas to burn it; the insulin then remains in the bloodstream, so you later get that "low blood sugar" feeling and a tendency to crave more sweets. The remaining insulin will turn into sugar in the bloodstream, and the sugar is stored as fat, otherwise known as triglycerides (refer to Chapter 8, page 69, to review the role of triglycerides in the body).

Our bodies have not evolved into machines that run endlessly on the many types of simple carbohydrates, processed starches, and sugar-rich foods that remain the trend in the American diet today. People are perplexed when their body wears down. Simply put, these foods create an energy deficit, and leave the body with nothing to work with except for the immediate synthetic rush you feel as the sugars flood the bloodstream.

Sugar is also the culprit for creating candida and yeast in the body, which is a condition that most people have but don't realize it. **"Candida Albicans"** are yeast infections often known as <u>Thrush</u>. A majority of Candida arises from the use of antibiotics, birth control pills, cortisone and many other commonly prescribed drugs. The problem begins when yeast (Candida) overgrows in the intestinal or urinary tract. As the Candida flourishes, the good bacteria, or flora, which lives in our intestines, are killed off. Eventually, the yeasts prevail, causing immune deficiency, fungal formation, skin problems, mood swings, PMS, depression and many more.

Sugar is also very acidic to the body, which throws off the acid and alkaline balance, which your body is trying to maintain. (See chapter 13 "Acid vs. Alkaline")

The hidden killer

Sugar is hidden in most of our processed foods. For instance, cereals that claim to have nutritional benefits often contain more sugar than any other ingredient. Ice cream is 50 percent sugar. Sugar is hidden in peanut butter, pickles, condiments, spaghetti sauce, baby food, salad dressings, canned fruits and vegetables, fast foods, and in all cured meats such as bacon and lunchmeats. Soda pop and powdered beverages retain 95 percent of their calories from sugar. One serving of a fruit flavored gelatin (which is supposed to be a lighter, weight-loss dessert), has 52 percent more sugar than a brownie! Read labels carefully. Sugar also appears under the names of sucrose, dextrose, maltose, lactose, and corn syrup.

Artificial Sweeteners

There are various "sugar-free" sweeteners available on the market today, most of which should be avoided and better yet banned from production. The **harmful** sugar substitutes are commonly known as:

- Aspartame (Equal, NutraSweet Sweet N' Low)
- Sucralose (Splenda),
- Saccharin High Fructose Sweeteners
- Refined Sugars and Acesulfame-k (Sunette, Sweet & Safe, Sweet One)

Let's explore these "Natural Sweetener Imposters" and see if you aren't appalled.

Aspartame

When you see "sugar-free" or "Sweetened with NutraSweet Sweet N' Low", or "Sweetened with Equal" on a food label, or if the ingredients include aspartame, a red flag should start waving.

Aspartame is an artificial sweetener synthesized from two amino acids: phenylalanine and aspartic acid with methanol (wood alcohol). It is used to sweeten unheated diet foods, diet beverages and powdered sugar substitutes. Recent European research shows that ingesting aspartame leads to the accumulation of formaldehyde in the brain, other organs, and tissues. Formaldehyde has been shown to damage the nervous system, immune system, and cause irreversible genetic damage in humans. Apartame has thus been linked to brain chemistry changes, tumors, behavior changes, headaches, depression, seizures, hives, vision problems, and menstrual difficulties. Researchers also found that foods containing aspartame, when consumed by women during pregnancy, have had an adverse affect on fetal brain development. Aspartame has also been linked to Alzheimer's disease.

An extremely large number of toxicity reactions have been reported to the FDA and other organizations. However, the FDA has repeatedly chosen to ignore this evidence. A recent report, just one of many, states that, "Of the 166 studies felt to have relevance for questions of human safety, 74 had Nutrasweet industry related funding and 92 were independently funded. One hundred percent of the industry funded research attested to aspartame's safety, whereas 92% of the independently funded research identified a problem." (Survey of Aspartame Studies: Correlation of Outcome and Funding Sources, by Ralph G. Walton, M.D., Chairman *of* The Center for Behavioral Medicine*)*

Third party studies also found that the chemicals, which the sweetener aspartame breaks down into, could be up to 50 times more toxic in humans than in rodents. Is this "sweetener" something that you actually want to ingest if given a choice? You have a choice, and I recommend that you just say no.

Sucralose (Splenda)

Let's talk about Splenda, otherwise known as Sucralose, also marketed by Johnson & Johnson under the catchy phrase, "It's made from sugar so it tastes like sugar". Splenda sales have far surpassed those of any other artificial sweetener. This "chemical" has monopolized the "Sugar-free" market behind the premise that it is a calorie-free natural sweetener. There is not one piece of evidence that can substantiate those claims!

Is Splenda a natural sweetener?

Read here and you be the judge: Splenda is a chemically altered version of sucralose. Sucralose, by itself, starts off as a sugar molecule. Splenda is produced by the process of morphing sucralose into a synthetic chemical through many stages in the laboratory. This new "Natural Sweetener" is actually made by combining sugar molecules with three times as many chlorine molecules. This new type of sugar molecule, known as a fructo-galactose molecule, does not occur in nature and therefore your body does not possess the ability to properly metabolize it. Hence, the FDA is falsely claiming that sucralose passes through the body unabsorbed. Since your body can't metabolize it, the chemical remnants are stored throughout the body. Sucralose consumption is equivalent to ingesting tiny amounts of chlorinated pesticides.

According to Dr. Joseph Mercola, as of 2005, only six human trials, totaling 36 people, have been conducted on Splenda. The only long term studies (a whole 3 months long) done on Splenda were after the FDA had already approved the artificial sweetener. Of the entire population, 36 people is not a large enough sample to guarantee safety, but the FDA's usual guidelines of what is safe for human consumption, and what is not does not fall into JGE's guidelines by a long shot. What is even worse is that the longest trial lasted only four days and they were looking at sucralose in relation to tooth decay, not human tolerance. Furthermore, because Splenda is only a food additive and not a drug, the number of studies required to receive FDA approval is substantially less than a drug. A scary fact is that no actual Long-Term Human Research has been done on this commonly ingested chemical.

In the same way that Splenda was marketed with few studies proving any safety, few studies were conducted on aspartame and saccharine. Studies didn't really begin until the negative health effects of aspartame and saccharine began to rise, raising alarm and provoking investigations. According to the Sucralose Toxicity Information Center, health side effects include shrunken thymus glands, enlarged liver and kidneys, decreased red blood cells, aborted pregnancy, diarrhea, reduced growth rate, and there are others. Also be aware that Splenda is found in about 3,500 food products and surprisingly many products do not list Splenda/Sucralose as an ingredient. Demand now, the labeling and research of this chlorinated chemical sweetener. Splenda is not sugar, is not natural, nor has it been proven safe!

*For further information and documented research, refer to: www.holisticmed.com and www.mercola.com .

Food Additives

The average American consumes almost 150 pounds of food additives per year, making it a multi-billion-dollar food processing industry. This breaks down to about 130 pounds of sugar and sweeteners, 10-15 pounds of salt, 5-10 pounds of "enriched" vitamins, flavors, preservatives, and colored dyes. There are about 12,000 other chemicals that contaminate our food during the various stages of growth, harvesting, packing, shipping and food preparation.

Natural and Artificial Flavors... A majority of these food additives, flavorings and preservatives, are masked behind the names "Artificial Flavors" and "Natural Flavors". Most processed and packaged foods, some of which can be found at health food stores, have over 300 unnatural chemicals hidden inside. How is that possible when these harmful substances are not listed on the ingredient label? Unfortunately, the FDA has allowed companies to add hundreds of toxins and chemicals under the code names, "Artificial and

Natural Flavoring". Try to avoid the product if you discover either of those terms, usually listed at the bottom of the ingredient list.

What is MSG? It stands for Monosodium Glutamate. This chemical has been called a preservative, but it is actually a taste enhancer, significantly modifying the flavor and taste of the food. If a food has gone bad, MSG can trick your taste buds so that you think it is still nourishing and fresh. Not only could you be eating rotten food, but it has also been proven that MSG can create harmful side effects. It can damage and create an imbalance in the body's cardiac, gastrointestinal, circulatory, muscular, and neurological systems. Eating MSG can lead to respiration, hyperactivity, vision, skin and urinary tract conditions.

When reading labels note that the following ingredients **always** contain MSG:

❖ hydrolyzed protein
❖ sodium cassenite
❖ yeast extract
❖ yeast nutrient
❖ maltodextrin
❖ autolyzed yeast
❖ textured protein
❖ calcium cassenite
❖ yeast food
❖ hydrolyzed oat flour

These ingredients **often** contain MSG:

❖ Malt extract
❖ Malt flavoring
❖ Bouillon
❖ Barley malt
❖ Broth
❖ Stock
❖ Flavorings
❖ Artificial flavorings
❖ Natural flavorings
❖ Natural beef flavoring
❖ Natural chicken flavoring
❖ Natural pork flavoring
❖ Seasonings

These ingredients **could** have MSG:

❖ Whey protein
❖ Trula yeast
❖ Carrageenan

- ❖ Smoke flavor
- ❖ Soy protein isolate
- ❖ Soy protein concentrate
- ❖ Whey protein concentrate
- ❖ Vegetable gum
- ❖ Added enzymes
- ❖ Corn syrup
- ❖ Pectin

Note: Soft Drinks, candy, and chewing gum can also be sources of hidden MSG

Have you ever heard the expression, "I feel full, but not full of the taste"? MSG is the culprit. Fast food restaurants use it for this very purpose -- it keeps you coming back for_more! It is suspected that the binders used for medications, nutrients and supplements for both prescription and non-prescription drugs, as well as drugs administered intravenously, may also contain MSG. MSG is even used in cosmetics, shampoos and hair conditioners -- especially those that contain hydrolyzed proteins or amino acids. Reactions to MSG may occur immediately after contact, or as much as 48 hours later. Some people react to very small amounts of MSG while others react only to large amounts or excessive usage. Why take the chance when you have a choice not to?

Irradiation

After World War II, the chemical industry needed to find new markets for its chemicals, so they expanded into food production. The industry's blind obsession for profits left little to no conscious consideration of how the chemicals would affect our health, the land, animals, and the environment as a whole. Government regulation expanded to issue tighter controls. The U.S. Department of Agriculture and the Department of Energy chose irradiation as a way to reduce the pesticides and toxic chemicals used to protect and preserve food. It is important that we are aware of this twisted unnatural measure that has been common practice for going on fifty years!

Irradiation, which uses high doses of gamma rays, kills insects and other pests in produce, kills the bacteria in meat, prolongs shelf life (processed foods), and delays ripening of fruits and vegetables. Irradiation is used most commonly on pork, fruit, spices, and vegetables. Choose foods labeled non-irradiated and organic. Avoid as many commercially processed foods as possible.

The U.S. Food and Drug Administration refuses to believe that irradiation produces foods that are carcinogenic; increasing the possibility of leukemia, liver cancer and kidney disease that may manifest as much as 20-30 years later. Irradiated food causes dangerous changes in human physiology as well. More immediate effects are lower birth weights and white blood cell and chromosome changes. Irradiation alters the protein structure of the food, decreases the vitamins and damages the enzymes. Irradiation destroys up to 80 percent of vitamins A, B, C, D, and K, while vitamin E is almost completely destroyed.

Not only is it harmful -- it doesn't work! Irradiation may kill the bacteria, but it cannot destroy the toxins produced by bacteria. These bacterial byproducts are deadly, cancer-causing agents that remain alive and well. Irradiated food contains free-radicals, which form new and dangerous chemical compounds in the food, such as benzene, hydrogen peroxide, and formaldehyde.

Free-radicals are actually forms of oxygen that have gone through excessive reactions. These destructive reactions occur when a free radical is created that has lost one electron, becoming unstable. To become stable again, the free-radical attaches to anything close by, like healthy cells. The healthy cell has now become oxidized and a new free radical cell has been born. The result is a chain reaction of free-radicals causing disease, mutation of the DNA, degenerative conditions and aging.

Table Salt

Sodium chloride (table salt) is concentrated and is a very unbalanced source of sodium. Common table salt lacks many trace minerals. In order to make salt white, it is washed many times, and in this process the valuable trace minerals are lost. Now, the salt is no longer a whole food. Following this refining process, the minerals are removed and sold to the chemical industry, or to pharmaceutical companies to make dietary supplements.

Food becomes deficient and can even become toxic when ingredients are removed from it. This is what happens with salt. Without the other minerals to balance it, salt becomes deadly when consumed excessively—as in the typical American diet. Salt is the most common preservative used today. Many foods are laced with a type of non-whole food salt—especially fast foods. French fries, milk shake beverages, sauce mixes, canned foods, and cured meats are major sources of salt.

Why do our bodies need "whole" sea salt?
A healthy, active lifestyle demands a reasonable salt intake. In the uterus, an embryo grows more than three billion times its conception weight in the salty environment of amniotic fluid. From the time of conception we are never without a need for salt. Our bodies contain three internal oceans that closely resemble the ionic balance of ocean water—the blood plasma, the lymphatic fluid, and the extra-cellular fluid. Each one of these complex solutions surrounds our cells and circulates through our bodies. Ocean salt contains all of the precious salts that our bodies require and it is because of these minerals that salt is a necessity.

Celtic Sea Salt and Himalayan Salt are two of the few salts I have found that contribute to a healthy body. Unlike other "sea salts," these salts have all of the necessary minerals and nutrients intact. Nothing has been extracted, so therefore these products are a whole food.

Genetically Modified Foods

Genetic engineering technology focuses on the manipulation (blocking, adding or scrambling) of the genetic material inside the cells of living organisms to block undesired or add desired traits. For example, researchers have been able to create a soybean with fertilizer and pesticides inherent in the seed. Be aware that hundreds of vegetables, fruits, grains and legumes are now being genetically modified, which is why it is so important to buy organic & "Non-GMO" labeled foods.

The jury is still out on exactly what the side effects could be from eating GMO foods, but our view is that any food that is altered from its natural state is going to be viewed as a foreign substance by your body, and there is no way to predict how each one of our bodies could potentially react to a food that has been genetically altered. Therefore, why even take the risk if there are companies and farms that are willing to make the extra effort not to take risks with you and your families' health?

We have detailed the dangers of consuming processed foods, and how a food loses more nutritional value as it is taken further from its natural state. A genetically modified food can be considered even worse than a food processed in hydrogenated oil and transfats because it not only is altering the chemical makeup of the food, but it is altering the food on a cellular level. Once again, why take risks when there are companies who have ethical standards in place that do not allow them to compromise your health? What can we do as consumers? We can support organic farms as well as state and federal legislation that require GMO farms to insulate their practices so as not to contaminate non-GMO farm fields. We can also demand that every food product on the market labels whether they are knowingly using genetically modified seeds or respective ingredients in their products or produce.

When you buy products that contain soy, rice, corn, canola seeds and wheat, or purchase fresh produce, be sure to read the label to determine whether the product has been genetically modified. Food manufacturers are not required to label whether their product has been genetically modified so if the label does not read, "Non-GMO, then you must assume that the food has been genetically modified. "Since genetically engineered soy and corn are used in many processed foods, it is estimated that over 70 percent of the foods in grocery stores in the U.S. and Canada contain genetically engineered ingredients."

Organic and GM Farms: An impossible coexistence?
If a product or produce is labeled "organic", is it guaranteed to be Non-GMO? Unfortunately the answer is no. The coexistence of GM and organic farms has become a great concern. There are hundreds of organic farms operating next door to where GM crops are being produced. The potential for plant seeds from the GM crops to be transported by wind is clear and present, and can contaminate and blend in with the organic seeds. Sadly, the major backers of GM farms are not responding to this serious issue, and have actually turned the blame on non-GM farms in some cases, actually claiming that because the GM seed has been found on a respective Non-GM farm, albeit in small quantity, the Non-GM farm has to pay a licensing fee to the GM producer. This is a serious problem, and one that is only growing worse as more and more Non-GMO and GM farms are operating in the vicinity of the other.

The OFRF, Organic Farming Research Foundation conducted a survey amongst organic farmers, which states, "The OFRF survey found that 27% of respondents have had a GMO test either requested or required by an organic certifier or a buyer." Erica Walz, OFRF survey coordinator, says, "Farmers who live in Midwestern states, where the majority of GM corn and soybeans are grown, reported significant impacts. When you look at farmers in Corn Belt states, it's a totally different picture. In these states, 70 to 80% of respondents reported negative impacts from GMOs." Iowa Governor Tom Vilsack has said that coexistence between GMO and organic should be a "national priority," and coexistence initiatives have been launched in several US states.

Processed Soy Products

Another caution is to avoid **Soy Protein Isolate**. This isolated protein was created for its ability to preserve, enhance flavor, and create a meat likeness, and is the most commonly used ingredient in many vegetarian meat-like foods such as:

- ❖ Soy protein shakes
- ❖ Veggie meats
- ❖ Veggie cheeses

"SPI" is the result of isolating soybeans, and processing them in an acid wash in aluminum vats. This process is not only highly toxic, but it creates a toxic food that is very acidic. This engineered toxin is more than likely worse for the body than eating the animal product itself.

CHAPTER
ELEVEN

<u>Animal Products</u>

Animal products are another staple to most people's diets. Over the years, there has been so much controversy over, "Should we or shouldn't we eat animals and their by-products?" I don't believe that there is only one right answer. I do feel strongly that we as a society place too much emphasis on animal products and focus less on plant-based foods. As I will discuss in this chapter, it is important to understand that our bodies were not intended for a high-animal diet. The bottom line is that meat and dairy is more difficult for all of us, regardless of our body type, to digest and always creates some unwanted acid and potentially lower energy. In chapter 13, Acid vs. Alkaline, you will learn how cooked and heavier foods need more enzymes from our body in order to break the food down. Cooked and pasteurized animal products qualify as enzyme-leeches, depleting our pool of enzymes.

I always tell clients, friends and family they must listen to their bodies as they experiment with different types and amounts of meat and dairy, because understanding the difference is the key to finding the balance. They then must decide for themselves if they need meat and/or dairy as part of their daily diet. Most feel more balanced with at least some fish and eggs, while others might lose stamina if they don't consume more animal protein. The one category I do feel is not necessary for any person/blood type/athletic status, etc, is cow-based dairy. Listen to what I have to say and make your own educated decisions. The categories are as follows:

Animal Products
- ❖ Dairy
- ❖ Meat
- ❖ Seafood

<u>Dairy</u>

Dairy products, as we know, come from animals. Furthermore, any medication given to the animal to maintain its health, or to cause it to grow bigger or grow faster, remains in their secretions. Dairy products, derived from secretions, can be saturated with tranquilizers, bovine growth hormones, antibiotics and diuretics. Studies done from 1987 to the present show increased levels of drugs and growth hormones in dairy products. The FDA revealed that 64 out of 82 drugs commonly given to dairy cows remain as residue in milk and other dairy products. ***You decide!***

If you choose to consume dairy products, be sure to buy only those from dairies that test their products.

Some of these are:
❖   Organic Pastures
❖   Alta-Dena Dairy
❖   Montebello Sanitary Dairy
❖   Natural Horizons
❖   Stuve's Natural and Stony Field Farms

These companies produce milk, yogurt, cottage cheese, sour cream, kefir, kefir cheese, crème fraiche, butter, frozen yogurt, and ice cream that have no detectable levels of veterinary drugs, antibiotics or genetically engineered bovine growth hormones.

Of the dairy products available today, the best choices are raw milk, raw butter, yogurt, and raw aged cheese. These foods have one thing in common - enzymes. Raw, un-pasteurized milk still contains enzymes to help your body break it down. Yogurt is a cultured food, which provides some enzymes and probiotic cultures such as acidophilus to aid digestion. Aged cheeses go through a fermentation process, providing more enzymes to aid in digestion. I am not recommending that you eat these regularly, but if you cannot eliminate dairy altogether, then try to choose from these raw products.

The other question we must ask ourselves is that apart from the contamination of dairy products, are any of these products actually good for your energy and daily nutrition? Mother's milk is essential for an infant's growth and development. Cow's milk is ideal for baby cows, helping them to grow from 100 to 600 pounds in about 6 months and supplying most of the nutrition that they need. However, cow's milk is not made for humans.

Cow's milk is high in fat calories (saturated fat), cholesterol, and lactose and is lacking in dietary fiber. Raised lactose levels can cause bowel problems such as diarrhea, stomach cramps, and intestinal gas. Dairy is one item that will eventually guarantee excess fat in the abdominal, hip and buttocks area. Another problem has to do with the mineral ratios in dairy, as with calcium to phosphorous, which are all completely out of balance for what our bodies need and can absorb. When cow's milk is ingested, the human body must leach calcium from our bones in order to balance the mineral ratios so that we can better absorb and eliminate the dairy. Because milk is so difficult to digest, the body assimilates only small levels of the calcium and protein that the cow milk industry claims you receive in abundance.

Even milk that is labeled "low fat" or "non-fat" is hard to digest. When fat is removed from milk products, the relative levels of protein and lactose are increased. Raised protein levels increase the likelihood of developing allergies and can actually cause calcium deficiency. As a whole, dairy products are not the wonderful calcium and protein sources that we have been told they are. Simply put, dairy products don't provide that good energy the body needs. It actually creates the opposite.

The best source for animal milk and related products is from goats and sheep. Next to coconut water, goat milk is actually the closest food to a human mother's milk. It is very similar in mineral ratios to the human body and to that of human milk. Because the calcium to phosphorous ratio in goat's milk is proportionately mirrored to that of our bodies, calcium is not leached from our bones and we are better able to absorb the calcium and other minerals present. People who are allergic to dairy or have difficulty digesting it usually do fine on goat and sheep products. If a baby is unable to breast feed, usually the next best thing to give them is goat's milk, or a goat milk based formula combined with coconut water, hemp or almond milk.

So, we know now that milk is not actually a good source of calcium or protein. However, our bodies do require calcium. Calcium, along with all the essential minerals are absorbed most efficiently when consumed as part of a whole food listed in the chart below. There are supplements that can help you access this essential mineral if you need to supplement. (For recommended servings, see our Circle of Life Eating Guide)

Whole foods that are highest in digestible calcium include:

- ❖ Sprouted greens
- ❖ Chia seeds – 5x more than milk & provides 35% of RDA
- ❖ Nuts & Seeds (Sesame and hemp seeds, walnuts, almonds, etc.)
- ❖ Dried fruit
- ❖ Yellow and Green leafy vegetables (Kale, Collard Greens, Spinach, etc.)
- ❖ Green grasses
- ❖ Algae (especially Hydrilla)
- ❖ Sea vegetables
- ❖ Fruits (dates, papaya, mango, apricots, avocados, oranges, strawberries, etc.) Legumes
- ❖ Black strap molasses
- ❖ Whole grains (Quinoa, Millet, Brown Rice, buckwheat, Kamut, etc.)
- ❖ Fermented foods (miso, seed cheeses, grain drinks)

MEATS

Do I need to eat meat?

I want to start my answer to this frequently asked question by first explaining the difference between carnivorous animals and plant eating animals. Animals that are carnivores (meat-eaters) have very short digestive systems -- about three times the length of their torso. Their teeth are very sharp and serrated, which is good for tearing flesh. Their whole digestive tract, starting with the saliva in their mouth, is highly acidic for the breaking down of concentrated proteins. The meats they eat do not stay in their systems very long, because their bodies are made to assimilate those types of foods. Meat eating animals also have an enzyme known as uricase, which breaks down uric acid and enables them to eliminate huge amounts of cholesterol through bowel movements.

In contrast, humans, like other plant-eating animals, have very long intestines--about 8 to 12 times the length of their torso. This longer intestine gives us sufficient time to digest and extract vital nutrients found in plants. Most of our teeth are flat and designed for grinding, and our saliva contains an enzyme (amylase) that only aids in the digestion of complex carbohydrates found in plants. Our liver, unlike the meat eater, is able to process only a small amount of cholesterol, and we do not have the uricase enzyme found in carnivorous animals that helps to break down meat. When we eat meat, we lack the high acid content in our digestive system to break it down. Now, let me just make note, that while this contrast between meat-eating animals and humans is generally true, some people do produce more acid than others, which is why some feel fine after eating meat and others feel sluggish.

Some health professionals feel that those who have more acid in their blood tend to need more meat in their diet. The more acidic the body is, the easier it is to break down meat while the more alkaline the body is, the more difficult it is to break down meat. (Learn more about the acid/alkaline balance in Chapter 13). Even if you have a higher acid level in the blood, this should not be a free pass to eat a lot of meats. Eating too much meat can create too much acid in the body. Too much acid can create illness, low energy, weight gain, and disease, so make sure you eat a balance of alkaline foods such as plant-based, unprocessed foods. Also, since meat is usually consumed cooked, it lacks the enzymes compatible to our digestive systems. Meat sits in our digestive tracts and putrefies, forming bacteria and causing digestive diseases, as well as blocking the lining of the digestive tracts where our food is assimilated.

People have been led to believe that human protein is built by eating only animal protein. Actually, proteins are built from <u>amino acids</u>. When a carnivorous animal such as a lion eats a zebra, its digestive system is able to assimilate zebra protein and transform it into lion protein. How does the lion's body do this? The lion eats the zebra raw. The amino acid chains in the zebra's raw protein are easily broken down and re-assembled into the lion's protein, or amino acid chain. Likewise, meat in its raw state naturally possesses the necessary enzymes to completely break itself down. That is why a whale can swallow a whole live seal and let it sit in its stomach for a week while the seal actually breaks itself down, returning excess enzymes to its host. When meat is cooked, the amino acids are fused together and the protein becomes unusable. Have you ever noticed that meat eaters rarely eat other meat eaters? Lions, tigers and other flesh eaters must eat plant eaters to obtain the nutrition that their bodies need to survive.

Now I am not saying that you should go out and start eating raw hamburger and pork – just the opposite! I am saying that you do not need to eat animal products in order to get your protein because it is the amino acids you want, not the animal meat.

Plant eaters, or vegetarians, get their amino acids from fruits, vegetables, nuts, sea vegetables and grains, which are sources our digestive tract is biologically adapted to utilize. So to be specific, EVERY amino acid needed to build human protein can be found in fruits, vegetables, and sea vegetables, green super-foods such as spirulina, and sprouted seeds, nuts, legumes, and grains.

However, those who are on an all plant-based diet must be sure to eat a large variety of <u>RAW</u>, protein-based foods in order to secure the essential amino acids.

A note on E-Coli Contamination
Reports are continually revealing problems created by the contamination of meats with E-coli and other bacteria. E-coli is spread through the fecal contamination of meat during the slaughtering process. E-coli usually linger on the surface of the meat. The bacteria are spread further after the hamburger is ground and mixed. Our health officials tell us that in order to kill the E-coli bacteria, we must cook the meat at 155 degrees Fahrenheit or above until it's well done—implying that if cooked properly, the meat is healthy and nutritious. This is an odd way to treat the problem, when the safeguards should start at the farm.

E-coli is not limited to meat, it has been found in various plant crops, such as spinach and lettuce. It can and has been the result of unclean water that is laden with fecal matter from pigs and other animals. Unfortunately we are all susceptible to E-coli contamination. E-coli contamination is definitely more common amongst meats, but can easily spread to plants and other crops which come in contact with contaminated water. Unfortunately, there is nothing we can do to keep from coming into contact with e-coli, but what I want you to know is that eating meats, especially those from fast food outlets does put you at a greater risk for e-coli bacteria, simply because of the lack in standards and quality of meat in many of these chains.

If you are going to eat meat...

As discussed in Chapter 11, the growth hormones, antibiotics and pesticides that animals consume and/or are injected with, should be enough to get our attention. Many of our cows, chickens and fish develop sores and cancerous growths that are cut out and the remaining "good" meat is sold for human consumption. Why risk the short term and long term health of yourself and your family for the sake of a protein that you can obtain from organic alternatives? This is a free society and all of you are autonomous individuals. Nobody can tell another person how to eat. It is a lifestyle choice, and it does not have to be a stressful one. If you are going to eat meat, be aware of the affect you are having on your energy and overall health, practice moderation, and cut down the risk of toxic transfer by choosing organic, free-range, and hormone free products.

Be sure to buy organic and eat more fish and white meats. The contamination in the non-organic commercial meat industry is so out of hand; it's not worth the risk. Also make sure to take digestive protein enzyme supplements to aid in digestion. (See pg. 133 for enzyme supplement recommendations)

How much protein do we need in our diet?

First, let me clarify the myth that if we don't eat meat, not only will we be protein deficient, but we will also become weaklings with underdeveloped muscles. Wrong! Check out some of the strongest animals in the world -- silverback gorillas, for instance. This fantastic species is three times our size and thirty times our strength. They live on bamboo leaves and fruit and can easily overturn a car! Do you want vibrant living strength or would you prefer being sleepy and lethargic, trying to digest high quantities of foods that are more difficult to digest?

Next, let's try to set some guidelines for how much protein your body actually requires.
The average person generally needs about 30-50 grams of protein daily. A good scale to go off of is about ¼-½ gram of protein daily for every pound you weigh. For example, if you weigh 120 pounds, you would be healthy with 30 to 50 grams of protein daily. The FDA conservatively recommends up to 55 grams daily to give a "margin of safety" for those who might need more protein in their diet.

Protein requirements can fluctuate, depending on individual needs. For example, athletes, weight lifters and those recovering from a surgery may need 80 or more grams of protein daily. Most Americans consume too much protein daily, 100 grams or more – largely in the form of cooked meats.

What are some of the specific foods that I can eat in order get my complete proteins if I don't eat meat at least once or twice a day?

Sprouted seeds, grains, and legumes are complete proteins? As we discussed earlier, the proteins that we, as plant-eaters, can assimilate, are found in fruits, vegetables and sprouted seeds, nuts and grains. Other sources high in proteins are pumpkin seeds, chia seeds, hemp seeds, legumes such as tempeh, adzuki, lentils, garbanzos, pinto, and black beans. Vegetables high in protein include artichoke, asparagus, fresh bamboo shoots, green vegetables, green leafy vegetables and vegetable greens. The sprouted grains highest in protein are rye, brown rice, and quinoa, amaranth and whole wheat.

It can be confusing and sometimes discouraging when trying to decide whether your body needs animal products, especially when you might be averse to eating animal products for reasons beyond how it affects your body. As I've said time and again, our bodies have a unique balance that must be achieved for health and daily energy to be optimal, and to prevent malnourishment in all forms.

At one time, I had cut out all fats and meats from my diet, thinking that was the answer to perfect health. After many years, I became imbalanced, low in energy, and stopped producing a balanced number of hormones. My body began craving raw fats (by the tablespoon-full), fish and goat cheese. It took me one year, but after first eating generous portions of raw fats such as coconut oil, nuts, seeds, avocados, and flax oil on a daily basis, I was finally able to introduce salmon into my diet. The result was that my body came alive and I couldn't eat enough salmon and other types of fish for the first couple of months. My body then fell into balance. I now eat fish, organic eggs and goat cheese in moderate amounts. I listen to my body, and have these animal products when my body asks for it.

My personal diet now includes mainly plant-based foods (eating about 70-80% raw foods), combined with wild fish about once a week. I generally eat organic eggs once a week. I eat raw goat cheese often and occasionally goat yogurt or kefir. You could say I am a vegan who also eats some fish, eggs, and goat products. My diet changes weekly, sometimes I don't want any animal products and some weeks I need more. Listening to my body has been my greatest tool. Like I have said, there is just not one right way of eating, just healthy guidelines and tips to follow!

One more thing... If you are deciding to become vegetarian, but don't eat a variety of all of the plant-based foods we have recommended, then you may need to have some fish and goat milk products so that you don't become mineral and amino acid deficient. Being vegetarian does not mean simply removing meat and/or dairy and then eating everything else available. We have seen some very unhealthy and/or overweight vegetarians and vegans because they eat a diet of processed foods full of refined flours, sugars, additives and processed oils, while forgetting to eat the high nutrient plant foods including raw and sprouted foods, sea vegetables, green grasses, and eating a large variety of vegetables, high protein grains, and legumes.

SEAFOOD

Is seafood a healthier alternative to other meats?

Fish is generally very friendly to our bodies, easily absorbed and very nutritious. Most people that cannot handle meat such as beef, pork, fowl, and game, have no problem with digesting fish. I know many vegans and vegetarians, who after many years of eliminating meat, incorporate fish into their diet and experience balance and satisfaction. Eating fish 2-3 times per week is a very healthy practice.

Fish is an ideal food, providing high quality protein (all of the essential Amino Acids), and Omega-3 Fatty Acids (EPA and DHA). As we discussed in Chapter 8, foods such as seafood, which is high in these Omegas, is crucial for reducing cholesterol (LDL) built up in the arteries, reduces inflammation in the body, stimulates the brain, balances the hormones, lowers blood pressure, and provides overall sustained good energy when prepared with natural alternatives.

Some of the most nutritious fish includes salmon, tuna, halibut, sea bass, cod, and trout. Salmon is probably the best seafood source of Omega Fatty Acids. Salmon is also high in iron, Vitamin A, B12, Calcium, Magnesium, Phosphorus, Potassium, and of course the essential Amino Acids. I like to eat salmon at least once a week, depending on my body's needs.

Fish is only as clean and healthy as the water it comes from. Make sure that you buy seafood labeled "Wild" and never "Farmed". Wild fish is least likely to possess as many toxins.

Mercury levels are a valid concern. Mercury stored in fish is usually found in the form of methyl mercury (the organic form). Unfortunately, it attaches easily and tightly to the protein tissue in fish.

Levels of mercury in fish are dependent on 4 main factors:

- ❖ The mercury content in the water
- ❖ Size of the fish
- ❖ A fish's lifespan
- ❖ Whether or not the fish has gills

Generally, the larger the fish, the higher levels of mercury stored. A fish that is higher on the food chain tends to eat a large variety of other fish. That large fish will absorb the smaller fish's mercury-laden protein. Fish types that live longer naturally absorb more mercury during their lifetime. As they age and grow larger, they are more likely to eat larger fish with higher mercury concentrations. Lastly, fish with gills are able to circulate clean water through their body and eliminate unhealthy toxins and wastes. Fish without gills don't have a built-in filtration system and are more likely to store toxins.

The body is capable of dealing with small amounts of mercury and it is normal to find trace amounts in the blood stream. As long as high-mercury fish are eaten sparingly, you shouldn't be alarmed. For those absorbing too much mercury through food, water, environment and injections, you may experience some common symptoms of mercury poisoning (fatigue, headache, memory loss and joint pain/ inflammation). Mercury toxicity can be very poisonous to the nervous system, has been linked to cancer, and can harm an unborn baby. If you are concerned about the mercury-levels in your body, the levels can be tested through blood and hair analysis.

Mercury levels are usually highest in the following fish.
Eat once every two weeks or less:

- ❖ Shark
- ❖ Swordfish
- ❖ Marlin
- ❖ King Mackerel
- ❖ Albacore Tuna
- ❖ Barracuda
- ❖ Seals
- ❖ Whales

Consume fish lower in the mercury chain 2-3 times per week:

- ❖ Wild Alaskan salmon
- ❖ Cod
- ❖ Herring
- ❖ Halibut
- ❖ Catfish

The next group of fish falls in the middle-range of mercury levels.

- ❖ Fresh Wild Ahi
- ❖ Sea bass
- ❖ Red snapper
- ❖ Trout
- ❖ Grouper

Smaller fish such as mackerel and sardines are extremely low in mercury due to their size. Most supplement companies who produce fish oils, generally use mackerel and sardines due to their low-mercury levels.

Tuna: Ahi vs. Albacore

Ahi tuna is also high in mercury but not as high as Albacore. Oddly enough, canned tuna is generally low in mercury because they use a lower-grade, smaller tuna fish, which does not store as much mercury. That doesn't mean that I am advocating canned tuna. Although lower in mercury, the tuna has been sitting in a can while absorbing the metals and chemicals. Plus, it is best to eat fish as fresh as possible. My recommendation on tuna is to only eat Wild Ahi, but try to limit this fish to no more than a couple of times per week.

Moderation | Awareness | Conservation

While the fish of the sea, lakes, rivers, and waterways are a wonderful part of our lives, providing us with nutrients like minerals, oils, and proteins, we know there is a balance that we must achieve for our children, grandchildren, and the generations beyond so that they all have the same healthy choices that we are fortunate to have the freedom to make today. The aboriginal Indians native to America believed intuitively that every action we take must be taken with seven future generations in mind. As the species at the top of the food chain, human beings have the highest responsibility to protect each level down the chain. I've often asked myself, "What can I do? How can I stop the speeding train representing the quest for profits throughout our lands and across our oceans?"

All of our actions should fall within a level of moderation since extreme behaviors generally lead to an imbalance. Our moderation in consumption and our choices not only help our bodies, but when practiced in union with other aware individuals, can help to correct the environmental balance.

The fishing industry has been operating within extreme parameters for decades because of the global increase in human populations, and the natural world is issuing desperate warnings. The oceans of today have reached a critical breaking point, and scientists are estimating severe shortages and even extinctions for many to most species of fish by mid century if industries across the world do not make significant changes in their practices in order to conserve the ecological balance of the oceans. My family and friends are trying to stay aware of what we as consumers can do to help influence the actions of irresponsible corporations who operate with profits in one hand, while the crucial hand of ecological balance sits idle. Just as with the body, every action creates a reaction, and a set of multiple consequences, so we must take a holistic approach that produces positive, balanced results. Balance in this case means providing the seafood that our bodies crave and the jobs that the industry provides people, but conserving the ecological health of the oceans that is more fragile than most of us realize.

We as consumers possess more influence than we might be aware of. The choices the masses make directly affect the profit margins of small, medium, and large food distribution companies. Mass media, especially the Internet, allows word to spread quickly. We must use these communication tools to free up the voices of many, and unite when companies decide that profits are more important than the health of the public and the Earth. Consumer activism is crucial during this time when change is no longer a choice but a requirement. It used to be about a person walking down to the beach and collecting clams, mussels, crabs, and lobsters, spearing a few tuna, or setting sail to net the catch for their family. These days, the majority of seafood is bought at a local market, and what a great amenity for our lives. When you visit the market, try to be aware of more than just the price. Where was the fish found, and what is the state of that species of that fish presently? Who is selling it, and is the company committed to conservation in balance with profits?

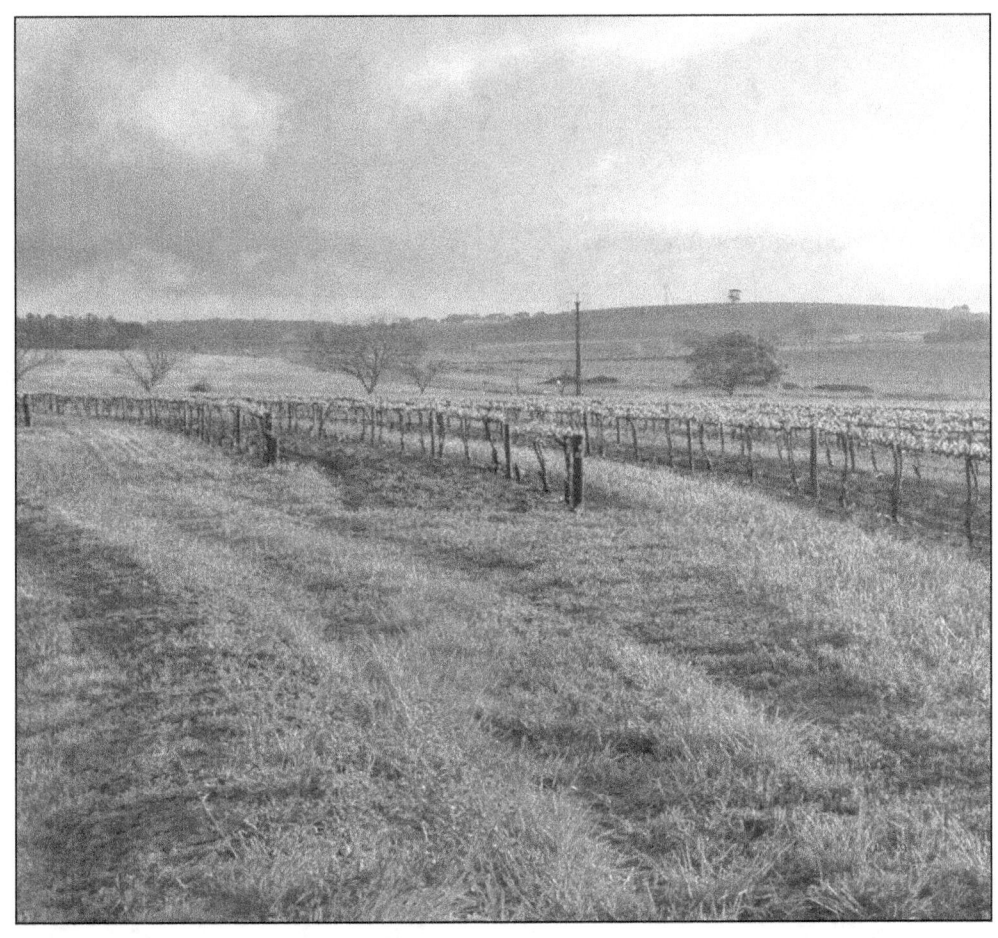

"In minds crammed with thoughts, organs clogged with toxins, and bodies stiffened with neglect, there is just no space for anything else."

~ Alison Rose Levy, "An Ancient Cure for Modern Life," Yoga Journal, Jan/Feb 2002

CHAPTER
TWELVE

Basic Food Combining

To understand the proper combining of foods, it is important to understand digestion. Food breakdown begins in the mouth with our saliva, which is why it is so important to chew our food, including juices, well.

Different types of digestive juices designed to digest specific foods exist in the stomach. Included with these digestive juices are your main digestive enzymes: **amylase,** for digesting carbohydrates; **lipase,** for digesting fat and **protease,** for digesting proteins. Some digestive juices are **acidic,** such as bile, and aid in breaking down acidic food like meat, dairy, nuts and legumes. Other digestive juices are more **alkaline**, for breaking down fruits, vegetables and grains.

The problem occurs when you are eating foods that require acidic digestive juices at the same time you are eating foods that require alkaline-based digestive juices. In these circumstances, the digestive juices often fight each other—denying proper digestion of either type of food. This causes stomach upset, gas, weight gain, and toxicity in your system. Obviously it is important to know which foods can be easily digested together.

Let's take a look at the types of foods that fall into the basic categories of proteins, starches, fruits, vegetables and liquids.

Proteins
- ❖ Flesh foods (beef, poultry, pork, fish) eggs and dairy products
- ❖ Nuts, seeds, dried legumes and dried peas
- ❖ Cooked and sprouted legumes
- ❖ Soaked, sprouted or fermented nuts and seeds and sprouted legumes. Because these are considered pre-digested foods, they are easier to digest than concentrated proteins; however, some people may still have problems mixing these with cooked starches.

Starches
- ❖ Breads, crackers, whole grain cereals, and foods made from grains, such as processed baked chips and tortillas
- ❖ Potatoes, corn, yams, winter squash and grains.
- ❖ Cooked, sprouted grains.
- ❖ Dehydrated sprouted-grain breads and crackers and sprouted grains are considered pre-digested foods that combine more easily with the other food groups.

Vegetables

Leafy greens, green and yellow vegetables, summer squash, green grasses, sea vegetables, all sprouted seeds and nuts, beets, buckwheat and sunflower greens, sprouts, cucumber, sweet peppers and carrots.

Fruits

- ❖ <u>Acid Fruits</u> - Oranges, limes, lemons, grapefruit, pineapple, pomegranates, strawberries and plums
- ❖ <u>Sub-acid Fruits</u> - Apples, apricots, berries, cherries, grapes, mangos, papayas, peaches, pears and plums
- ❖ <u>Sweet Fruits</u> - Bananas, coconut, dates, figs, dried fruit and persimmons
- ❖ <u>Melons</u> - Cantaloupe, casaba, crenshaw, honeydew and watermelon

Liquids

Water, fruit juices, fermented grain drinks, herb teas, nut, fruit and grain milks, vegetable juices, wheat grass.

Basic food combining guidelines

You don't have to be extreme with your food combining. I am just laying out the ideal guidelines. Some people's stomachs are more sensitive to food combinations while others are not. Experiment with my recommended combinations below, and see what gives you the best energy.

Recommended Combinations

Fruits, fruit juices, and fruit milks

- ❖ Should be eaten alone on an empty stomach.
- ❖ Eat fruit alone, about a half-hour before other types of foods, or two+ hours after
- ❖ Melons should be eaten alone
- ❖ Apples, tomatoes, and avocados are the only neutral fruits that can be eaten with grains, protein, vegetables and most food groups.

> ❖ **Almonds** are both in the protein and fruit categories. As a type of milk, we mix them with soaked and/or sprouted grain. Because almonds are also fruits, we grind them up and use them in raw fruit pie-crusts

Vegetables

- ❖ Can be mixed with proteins or starches, but never with fruits

Cooked proteins

- ❖ Can be mixed with cooked vegetables but never with fruits or cooked starches
- ❖ The biggest concern is animal protein. Try to avoid mixing animal products (meat and dairy) with any cooked starches.
- ❖ Raw or fermented proteins can be mixed with raw vegetables, sprouted starches, and dehydrated starches

❖ Even though soaked nuts, seeds, and legumes (raw or cooked), are a protein, they are okay to mix with starches as long as everything has been soaked and/or sprouted first

Cooked Starches
❖ Can be mixed with cooked vegetables, but never with fruit or animal protein.
❖ Raw, sprouted, or sprouted and dehydrated starches can be mixed with raw vegetables and fermented or sprouted proteins.

Super-foods
❖ Green and red super-food drinks (combination of green grass juices, sea vegetables, and algae or antioxidant-rich berries) are best when consumed on an empty stomach.
❖ Drink first thing in the morning and wait at least 15-30 minutes before consuming solid food. See chapter 16 for more details about my recommended super-food products.

Most liquids
❖ Drinks (juice, water, tea, etc.) should ideally be consumed 15-30 minutes before a meal and 30-60 minutes after a meal.
❖ Drinking water 15 minutes before a meal is fine and will help you to feel less hungry at your meal, but try not to drink with food.
❖ Vegetable juices and sprouted grain drinks can be mixed with raw vegetables and sprouted, or sprouted and dehydrated, grains.

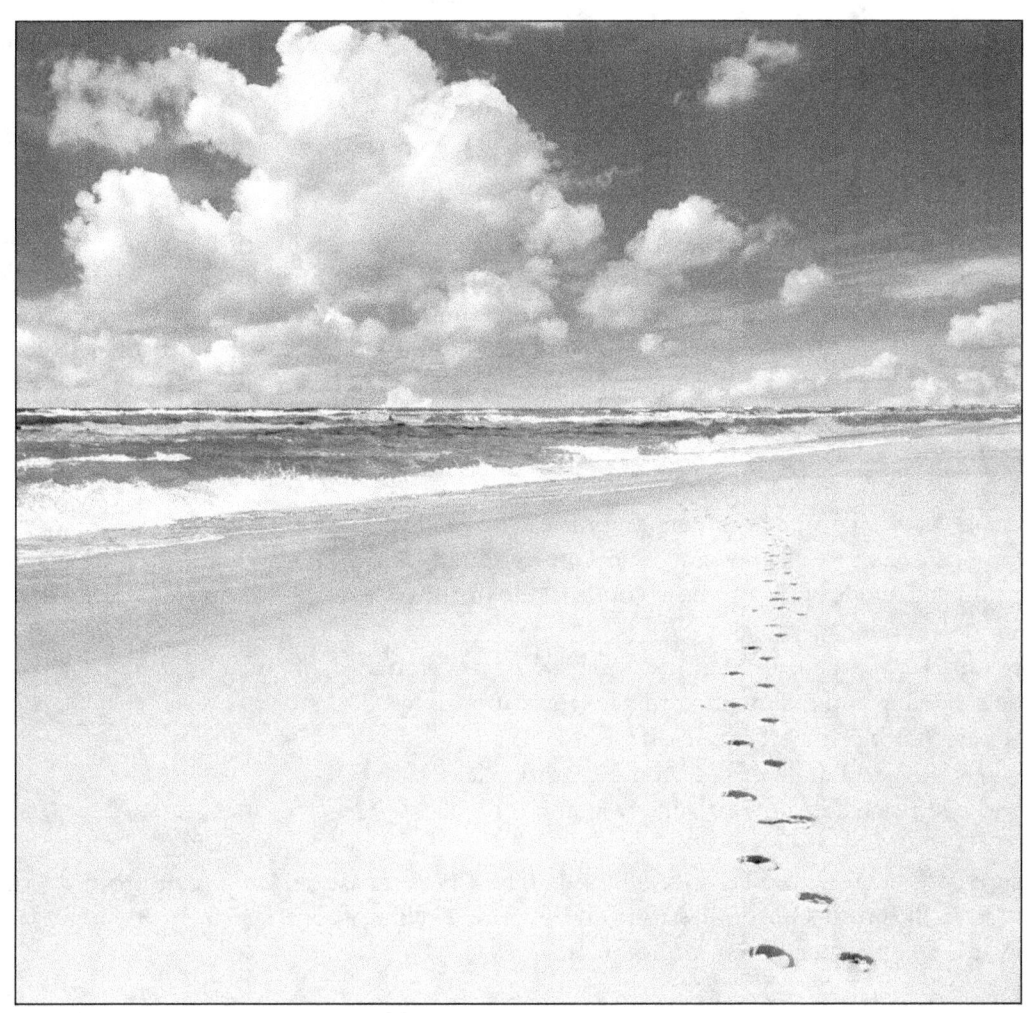

*"Health is a state of complete harmony of the body, mind and spirit.
When one is free from physical disabilities and mental distractions,
the gates of the soul open." ~ B.K.S. Iyengar*

CHAPTER
THIRTEEN

Acid vs. Alkaline

Whether your body is in an acid or alkaline state will determine the quality of life you will experience. You may have heard the term "Acidosis". This refers to the condition of your blood and having a PH that is too acidic. Acidosis is not one specific disease; it is the breeding ground for other diseases to develop and be nurtured, such as cancer, osteoporosis, heart disease, high blood pressure, arthritis, obesity, diabetes, allergies, kidney stones, premature aging, and many other degenerative diseases. It is possible to have Alkalosis (too much alkaline), however it is not very common. Over 90% of the population today is too acidic and has Acidosis.

It is important to have a complete understanding about Acidosis and develop an intense desire to change your lifestyle to become more alkaline and enjoy the benefits. The following topics will help you understand what is going on inside your body and how you can transform your quality of life. Let's explore:

- ❖ What does acid, alkaline and PH mean regarding my blood?
- ❖ Why is achieving and maintaining this balance important?
- ❖ How does your blood become acidic?
- ❖ How does the body deal with too much acidity (Acidosis)?
- ❖ How do you reach a healthy balance of being more alkaline?

PH is a measure of how much acid is in the blood. The PH is measured on a scale from 0 to 14 (0 = pure acid and 14 = pure alkaline). Our body strives to be more alkaline, about 7.3 - 7.4. A variant of as little as 2 full points towards acidity, such as 5.3, could be fatal.

There are two different types of acidic foods & alkaline foods. Most people are familiar with acid or alkaline foods, *which means how much acid or alkaline the food contains*. The second and more important is acid or alkaline forming foods, which means the PH condition which foods create in the body/blood after being digested and reabsorbed into the blood stream. This is what changes the body's blood PH levels. Acid-forming foods create an acid ash when completely burnt, while Alkaline-forming foods leave an alkaline ash when completely burnt.

The importance of reaching a balanced PH state in the body cannot be emphasized enough. If one truly cares about their quality of life, body, and spirit, then this should be taken very seriously. As mentioned previously, the acidic state is the root of most disease, sickness, and emotional/mental problems.

Scientists have found that cancer thrives in an acidic solution, while it is unable to survive in alkalinity. Just as an embryo grows rapidly and flourishes in the mother's womb surrounded by amniotic fluid, a germ grows quickly and strongly in an acidic environment. By creating an acidic state in our bodies, we are therefore encouraging disease and chaos to be created within. The truth is that germs are not the source of disease. We create our own harmful & polluted inner environment, which in turn allows the germs to multiply, feed and create their own pollution.

There are a few simple and common factors, which disrupt the alkaline balance:

Our thoughts, emotions and stress-levels are very strong factors that are often overlooked when trying to reach alkalinity. They physically create large amounts of acid in our blood when being experienced. *Your thoughts are creative and will have a physical manifestation.* This is a saying that is very true. Stress can cause serious breakdowns and problems within your body no matter how healthy you are eating. That is why stress-management and deep-breathing exercises are so important and can change the state of your body

All natural foods contain both acid and alkaline forming elements. In some foods, acid-forming elements dominate and vice versa. Such acid-forming foods include animal proteins, cooked oils, alcohol, pasteurized dairy, caffeine, refined/processed grains & carbohydrates, most cooked grains that haven't been soaked/and or sprouted first, and all cooked nuts & legumes that have not been soaked and/or sprouted first. (Refer to the Acid& Alkaline Food Chart, page 114).

Other prevalent factors induce an acidic state within us are: tap water, smog, radiation, pesticides, chemical preservatives, food dye, and additives.

Lastly, over-exercising your body can actually create an acid state in the body. When people are so concerned about losing weight and go to the gym 2-3 hours daily and are not losing the weight, they get frustrated and stressed. This state of being can create too much acid (lactic acid) in the body. Exercise regularly but moderately.

When the blood is overwhelmed with acid ash from foods and stressful emotions, the body relies on a few keys to neutralize acid:

When acid is present; the body must then absorb and neutralize it to become more alkaline. Luckily our bodies are designed with alkaline cell storages, which can soak up the acid to neutralize it. Unfortunately these cells can mutate and become abnormal cells because the acid, during the neutralization process, actually strips the negative charge surrounding the cells. This causes the cells to "glue" together and possibly form malignant/cancerous cells. Simply put, acid could be referred to as glue. Since there are only so many alkaline storages available at a time, the body must use other tactics.

Another tactic is for the body to produce fat cells, which absorb the acid and neutralize it. The unfortunate result creates many unwanted fat cells roaming the body. These cells eventually will lose their respective +/- charges, clump together, and move sluggishly, until they are stored in pockets. This creates excess body fat and lowered energy.

The veins and arteries are defenseless culprits of acidic blood. They are the transport system for the blood to flow throughout the entire body. If the blood running through a vein is highly acidic, a hole could be burned through the vein, allowing the acid to invade the rest of the body. To prevent this, the veins and arteries create and form plaque surrounding the inside walls. This plaque buffers the wall, not allowing the acid to burn a hole. Consequently this self-defense mechanism can be detrimental to one's health. Clogged veins and arteries are precursors to heart attacks, high blood pressure, and many other heart-degenerative diseases.

One last common method of protection is the muscles. Muscle tissues will also absorb and neutralize acid when there is excess for a long period of time. The unfortunate consequence here is that the muscles eventually become "flabby" because the muscle tissues are breaking down. People eating a very acidic diet to lose weight (high-animal protein) are very likely to lose more muscle tone quickly than one who is eating a balanced diet.

There are important steps one can take to reverse the acidic state:

First, purchase PH strips, which can be found at pharmacies or health food stores. It will have a chart to show you your PH number. Check your PH in the morning before eating. Normal is considered 7.3-7.4, however, above 7 is still considered healthy. The main concern is when your number shows 6.5 and below.

It is important to cleanse the body of toxins that have developed and taken residence over the years. Drinking alkaline water for one to two weeks can help to alkalize your system. Also drinking a "green drink" daily will add to your alkalinity and aid in the cleansing process, including, wheat grass, sea vegetables, chlorophyll, green grasses, spirulina, etc. These greens are one of the most alkaline foods. Kombucha Tea is very alkaline and is ideal for obtaining that ideal PH.

The target balance is to eat about 65%-75% alkaline-forming foods, 25%-35% acidic. Some alkaline-forming foods include fresh fruits, vegetables, fermented foods, raw soaked/sprouted nuts & seeds (almonds are the most alkaline), raw/un-pasteurized goat/dairy products, sprouted whole grains, tempeh, sea vegetables, etc.

Practice proper food combining. When you combine properly you reduce purifications in the body, thus creating a more alkaline condition.

Find the disruptive pattern or emotion that is creating stress in your body and work on reversing it. Try yoga, a walk, deep breathing exercises, meditation, or simply being aware of acid-causing emotions as they arise.

❖ **Kombucha Tea: A daily detoxifier, healer, and nutrient provider**
Let us share a health secret with you that has become a daily part of our lives…

The Kombucha culture is a colony of yeast and bacteria (the friendly type which naturally exists throughout our digestive tract), which makes it probiotic, detoxifying and energizing. Although often referred to as a mushroom, it is actually a symbiotic culture of bacteria and yeast. It helps build up immune systems, alkalize the body, fights yeast infections and helps joint problems.

Kombucha Tea is made by combining the culture with a mixture of black or green tea and raw sugar. The ingredients are then allowed to "ferment" for about 15-30 days. Kombucha tea has been used as a healing elixir, known as "Miracle Fungus" or "Cure-all", by the Chinese for over 2,000 years and has become increasingly popular over the past 4 decades.

Kombucha may not be the direct cure to a multitude of illnesses, but it works with your body to boost its natural ability to fight sickness and disease as well as bring a healthy balance back to your metabolism and organs.

The tea can be purchased at health food stores or made right at home. If the tea is bought, make sure the label says "Raw" and not "Pasteurized". The taste can produce a slightly sparkling drink that tastes like an apple cider or a wine cooler. Because Kombucha is fermented, there is alcohol in it, but there is less than 0.05%, which allows commercial producers to label it as "non-alcoholic". Sugar is used as part of the recipe but it is not used as a sweetener. The sugar is broken down and converted into different components of the finished drink.

So Drink up and enjoy the benefits!

Alkaline vs. Acid Food Chart

Personal Note: If your body is more alkaline then you are naturally in a higher state of consciousness. More Acidic – the more grounded and lower state of consciousness

Alkalizing Foods – Goal 65-75%

VEGETABLES
Garlic
Alfalfa
Artichoke
Asparagus
Avocado
Fermented Veggies
Watercress
Beets
Broccoli
Brussel sprouts
Cabbage
Carrot
Cauliflower
Celery
Chard
Chlorella
Collard Greens
Corn, raw
Cucumber
Dandelion Greens
Eggplant
Kale
Kohlrabi
Lettuce
Mushrooms
Mustard Greens
Dulce
Dandelions
Edible Flowers
Onions
Parsnips
Peas
Peppers
Pumpkin
Rutabaga
Sea Veggies
Spinach
Spirulina
Sprouts
Squashes
String Beans
Swiss Chard
Alfalfa
Barley Grass
Wheat Grass
Wild Greens
Nightshade Veggies

FRUITS
Apple
Apricot
Avocado
Banana
Cantaloupe
Cherries
Currants
Dates/Figs
Grapes
Grapefruit
Guava
Lime
Melons
Nectarine
Orange
Lemon
Lime
Mango
Peach
Pear
Persimmon
Pineapple
Plum
Pomegranate
Prune
Raisins
All Berries
Tangerine
Tomato
Tropical Fruits
Watermelon

PROTEIN
Sprouted beans
Almonds
Chestnuts
Tofu (fermented)
Flax Seeds
Chia Seeds
Flax Oil, cold-pressed
Pumpkin Seeds
Tempeh (fermented)
Squash Seeds
Sunflower Seeds
Millet
Sprouted Seeds
Raw Nuts-Soak 1st

Young Coconut meat

OTHER
Apple Cider Vinegar
Agar
Bee Pollen
Lecithin Granules
Probiotic Cultures
Green Juices
Veggies Juices
Fresh Fruit Juice
Organic Milk (Raw/un-pasteurized)
Mineral Water
Alkaline Water
Green Tea
Herbal Tea
Dandelion Tea
Ginseng Tea
Banchi Tea
Kombucha
Young Coconut Water

SWEETENERS
Stevia
Honey, Raw & pure
Yacon Syrup

**SPICES/
SEASONINGS**
Cinnamon
Curry
Ginger
Horseradish
Mustard
Chili Pepper
Sea Salt
Miso
Tamari
All Herbs
Coconut Aminos

ORIENTAL VEGETABLES
Maitake
Daikon
Dandelion Root
Kelp
Shitake
Kombu
Reishi
Nori
Umeboshi
Wakame

Acidifying Foods — Goal no more than 30% at most

REFINED FATS & OILS
Avocado Oil
Canola Oil
Corn Oil
Hemp Seed Oil
Lard
Olive Oil
Safflower Oil
Sesame Oil
Sunflower Oil

FRUITS
Cranberries

COOKED GRAINS
Rice Cakes
White Flour
Gluten
Whole Wheat
Amaranth
Barley
Buckwheat
Corn & products
Oats (rolled)
Quinoi
Rice (all)
Rye
Spelt
Kamut
Hemp Seed Flour

DAIRY
Cheese, Cow
Sour Cream
Cheese, Processed
Cheese, Goat
Cheese, Sheep
Milk
Butter
Cottage Cheese
Cream
Cream Cheese
Ice Cream
Margarine

NUTS & BUTTERS
Cashews
Coconut, dried
Brazil Nuts
Peanuts
Peanut Butter
Pecans
Tahini
Walnuts
All Roasted Nuts

ANIMAL PROTEIN
Beef
Carp
Clams
Egg Yolks
Fish
Lamb
Lobster
Mussels
Oyster
Pork
Rabbit
Salmon
Shrimp
Scallops
Tuna
Turkey
Venison
Processed & Smoked
  All Meats

PASTA (WHITE)
Noodles
Macaroni
Spaghetti

SWEETENERS
Sugar Cane
Sorghum Syrup

DRUGS & CHEMICALS
Chemicals
Drugs, Medicinal
Pesticides
Herbicides
Tobacco

ALCOHOL
Beer
Spirits
Hard Liquor
Wine

BEANS & LEGUMES
Black Beans
Chick Peas
Green Peas
Kidney Beans
Lentils
Lima Beans
Pinto Beans
Red Beans
Soy Beans
Soy Milk
Soy - Processed foods
White Beans
Rice Milk

OTHER
Distilled Vinegar
Wheat Germ
Potatoes
Soda
Caffeine
Coffee
Soda
Processed/Refined
Fried Foods
Shortening
Table Salt
Caffeinated Tea
Fruit Juice, Pasteurized
Yeast & Malt
Tap water

NEUTRAL LEANING TO ALKALINE FOODS:

Whole Grains sprouted/soaked
Cottage Cheese
Coconut
Goat Milk Cheese/Yogurt
Wild/Mercury & Hormone Free:
Fish
Acidic Nuts that have been soaked
Yogurt – Unsweetened
Almond Milk
Raw/Unpasteurized dairy
Raw/Cold Pressed Oils:
  MacNut, Almond, Grapeseed, Olive,
    Avocado, Safflower,
  Sesame & Sunflower
Whey
Egg Whites

CHAPTER
FOURTEEN

Weight Loss: From the Inside Out

Weight loss and gain is a wild dance; a complex process governed by the complexities of life. As such, the loss and gain of pounds is a fluid course just as material and emotional loss and gain are ever-changing.

Many individuals and companies have profited upon the promise of standardizing what is an extremely custom lifestyle solution. There is not one single body type. Thus, there cannot be a one-size-fits-all methodology, stratagem, or philosophy for achieving an ideal weight. Offering single solutions for weight management attenuates what is a broad and variable subject.

To be clear and fair, there are a multitude of programs, products and techniques that can absolutely help achieve short term weight loss. There are consistencies in our physical systems such as digestion, metabolic and hormone fluctuation that make it possible for certain tenets, strategies and tactics to apply to masses of individuals. These "programs", if properly calibrated for customization, can even deliver sustained results.

However, this chapter and this book are not about short term transitions, but are about transitioning to a lifelong, self-owned practice of natural living. The practice has to be a custom course that each of us purposely design, own, and adapt as we cycle through life. The working goal is a natural, sustained and fluid way of life rather than an artificial, short term approach based on narrow measurements such as calorie totals.

Your weight is just one important barometer to measure the results of a natural lifestyle design. In order to control weight fluctuation, you will benefit from establishing a combination of self-measurements such as how clear your mind is, and the tone and feel of your skin, the strength of your hair, muscle mass, joint health, and so forth. Measuring your health by your weight total alone is like measuring a book or movie by the title and not the actual parts that makes up the working whole. Weight management is one major part of your holistic and balanced approach to your health.

The first step in powering your natural transition that will result in natural weight loss is to understand how your body operates and what it needs for optimal energy. Progress and evolution require energy. Once you understand how to energize for your own lifestyle, you will be empowered to design a custom course that powers you with enough clean energy to propel your transition for life-long results.

Cause and Effect:
Weight gain is easy. If you eat too much and do not release that energy production through exercise, then you will gain weight. If the foods and beverages you are consuming are high in bad fats and other heavy, non-digestible ingredients, you will gain weight at a faster pace, and the weight will be based upon more visceral fat that is extremely difficult to lose.

Over-eating applies to healthy and unhealthy diets. Portion control is the absolute in any weight loss formula, and it is as critical to apply portion control when making your natural transition. It is true that you could eat larger portions of raw, nutrient dense food and not gain as much weight as if you were eating foods that are high in bad fats, but you will gain weight none the less. My standard ratio of raw, plant based foods to cooked foods is 70% raw / 30% cooked. This ratio is especially important when making incremental choices throughout your day with weight loss in mind.

Sustained Weight loss is more difficult because it is not so much a cause and effect of any one action such as eating less carbohydrates or more protein, but rather the result of careful adjustments in the orchestra of incremental choices we make every day from what we eat and drink, how much we eat at one sitting, what time of the day we eat, how fast we eat; how we combine food and drink; cleanse from the day before, and how we mix and blend all these choices with the other variables of life each twenty-four hour cycle.

Regardless of where you are in your transition, you must put in place tenets or behavioral codes to achieve a denominating synchronization between nutrition and exercise. This total integration works as a foundation so that you can continue progressing even when life is most challenging. It is that triangulation between your <u>orchestra of daily choices</u> along with time-managing <u>life variables</u> such as stress, sickness, sleep, children, balanced with the <u>daily fitness activities</u> you schedule each day that will ultimately determine your weight.

If you were to ask what is more important for losing weight—exercise or nutrition, my answer is that weight loss starts with nutrition because your consumption will regulate all of the functions of your body and mind and produce the energy to fuel exercise. When optimal nutrition is consistently integrated with daily exercise, you will gradually achieve your ideal weight and overall shape that you desire.

As you make your transition, examine your energy throughout the day. Where does it drop off? Are you just not performing the physical and mental functions at optimal capacity? Energy should be sustained. It should not fluctuate dramatically.

5+1

Let's dig in by redefining the "meal". A meal can be any type of beverage or food. It can be an apple. It can be an apple smoothie. It can be an apple pie. It does not have to have courses. I does need an appetizer, entrée or be eaten in any particular order. There are occasions of course where rituals and traditions require specific choices, but all I am saying is that in order to change our habits we must be open to customizing our own eating in a way that is outside the very linear American practice of breakfast, lunch and dinner, which doesn't account for all the activity in between.

Simply, there is not one size or choice required of any meal at any time of day. The choice and size of a meal depends on your energy demand at that time of day. The tactic is to keep from becoming too hungry at any given time while sustaining maximum energy.

The 5+1 approach is the one I follow and it is basically a practice that relies on preparing food ahead of time for a morning jumpstart followed by five "meals" from morning through to evening. The risk of course of having too many feedings is that there are more opportunities to overeat. This approach will only be effective if you exercise common sense portion control based on your energy demand.

What differentiates this approach is first, the definition of a *meal*, and second, that you are eating with a focus on energy rather than fullness. If you eat too much at any one sitting, your energy will drop because your body will be consumed by the process of digestion. As I said, a *meal* can be anything you put in your body regardless of the size. Each choice should directly relate to your energy demand on each respective day. To illustrate, a fifteen year old training for his wrestling team has a much different energy demand than a forty-five year old stuck at the office ten hours a day. It is all about keeping your energy in balance. It is also about making a natural transition with the healthiest choices for sustained, balanced living rather than a regimen that provides negative, nutrient weak foods that might be helping one lose weight, but is not providing positive energy.

This approach also empowers you to customize your diet through learning how to prepare your own meals ahead of time rather than depending on mostly pre-packaged products that might make you more dependent on them for your choices. The macro goal is to empower you to be your own nutritionist and your own chef so that you can lead an independent life and pass down those practices to your children and loved ones.

The +1 is to start every day with a green super-food drink for both detoxification and jumpstarting your metabolism and overall energy. I recommend adding a pure green Matcha tea for a boost. Your five meals will be consumed between 7a and 7p for maximum weight balance. You'll have to adjust your portions within that range to energize your exercise regimen. Everyone's schedule is unique so you'll have to find the right portion size for you based on your energy requirements each day. Keep in mind that the body requires a-lot less energy for an office job than an outdoor vocation with more movement. Apply your portions appropriately based on your energy requirements. If your portion control is in-balance with your choices during your natural transition—you will gradually reduce and eliminate excess fat and weight.

Next, I am going to give you the fundamental guidelines you need to be aware of when transitioning to a natural lifestyle while reaching your ideal weight. This is not a step by step program, or a particular kind of diet. They are fundamental rules to understand so that you can attribute your weight fluctuations to specific behaviors. You have the ability to adapt to these rules and adjust your behaviors that will determine whether reaching your ideal weight is one of the results of your natural transition.

15 Guidelines to an Ideal Weight through a Natural Transition

1) Simplify
Going natural and losing weight is about simplifying your diet to a more raw, plant based diet. Less really does equal more.

2) Go Natural
The more processed and dysfunctional a food is, the more difficult it is to digest. The digestive potential for a food is the bottom line, and far more defining than a food's calorie count. Simply, if a food takes longer to digest, it stores more readily as fat. Raw corn on the cob is in its natural state, while fried corn oil in a corn tortilla chip has been so processed that the body can't even recognize it as food and has a hard time

digesting it. Certain carbohydrates, such as refined white flour, or any processed flour, white rice, potatoes, corn and other starches tend to produce more insulin in the body. Even whole wheat flour can raise your insulin levels. The insulin transforms into glucose, or sugar, and when it is not used up, the excess is stored more readily as fat.

So when shopping for functional foods, try to avoid processed or packaged foods, which include chips, breads, pastas, and basically anything canned, boxed or bagged that has any added chemical ingredients including preservatives and unwanted additives.

There is a more flavorful, natural alternative for everything—yes, including butter and sugar! Refer to Chapter 19 on natural alternatives for all types of foods.

3) Cleanse
We discussed the importance of cleansing and detoxifying your systems in Chapter 3. Cleansing is important for weight reduction for multiple reasons. You have stored weight in the form of fat cells that have built up in your colon and in visceral areas, primarily around the abdominals and glutes. Fat stores in all your systems including your tissue, skin, around your organs and it all leads to unnecessary toxic weight.

Think of cleansing as the ignition for putting your body in the position to lose weight. I recommend initiating a daily cleanse of a morning drink and a longer 3-day juice cleanse one time a month. The daily cleanse is for life, while the 3-day cleanses are for ignition and for occasions when you know you are clogged. If you are significantly over weight, or feel overly toxic, you might deploy a longer cleanse, and augment your cleansing by including a series of colonics.

I've included a three-day or eleven-day cleanse outlined in Chapter 3. You may also choose a series of colonics for faster weight-loss. I recommend consulting your doctor before undertaking any type of dramatic cleanse, especially if you have existing health issues.

4) Do not starve
Eating is important for weight loss even when you are cleansing. If you don't nourish with any substance over a period of days, you risk slowing down your metabolism, which is what you don't want. If you don't eat for more than 3-4 hours, your metabolism might begin to slow, which creates the environment for storing fat. The body basically thinks that you might not eat again so it creates stores as a contingency.

5) Recognize empty calories
While calorie counting plays a part, it is not the only measurement that we should be using. Measuring calories focuses on the quantity of daily food intake, but not necessarily the quality of the food you are consuming. Below here are just five common examples of misconceived foods that are promoted as "weight loss foods". These are foods that are low in calories but provide minimal if any nutrition and can actually add in weight gain and toxicity:

   a. **Sugar:** A food made with mainly sugar, flour and spices might be low in fat or even fat free, but once your body absorbs this "food", it becomes extremely fattening and actually pulls nutrients away from the body. ***Compare*** that to a piece of raw fruit that of course naturally has sugar and calories but the fruit breaks itself down in your stomach and provides nutrients.

b. **Rice Cakes:** Low in calories but also low in nutrients. Plus it is high on the glycemic index which can raise your blood sugar levels causing a rise in glucose production and fat storage. *Compare* that to a sprouted tortilla that is a bit higher in fat and calories but is high in protein, healthy grains, and lots of fiber – it fills you up much longer and satisfies the body without creating a rise in insulin levels.

c. **Chemical sugar-free sweeteners** such as aspartame, Splenda, Sweet 'n Low, Equal, etc – They have no sugars and/or barely any calories but actually cause the stomach to store fat in the abdominal area plus damages brain cells, the central nervous system and more. Watch out for the sugar-free sodas – they are worse than the regular sodas and beverages. *Compare* that to Stevia that is also a low calorie and sugar-free product but is an actual food extract from a plant that is nutritious, healing and safe without causing the body to produce fat.

d. **A label that reads Fat-free on a premade and packaged food**: This is a warning flag because these foods are generally packed with sodium to replace the flavor, chemical flavor enhancers, sugar-free sweeteners or even regular sugar and processed white flour. All of these food additives can be low in calories but provide no nutrition and cause more harm to the body. *Compare* that to an organic already made meal that has few ingredients, no chemicals, preservatives or natural/artificial flavorings, higher in fiber, low in sodium and made without milk and cheese.

6) Food Combining

Understanding food combining principles are an important part of weight loss. Different types of foods do not digest well with other foods. Certain digestive juices cancel out others, creating digestive problems that can lead to the storage of fat. (See Chapter 12 for more on food combining).

Generally, combine meats only with vegetables: carbohydrates can be combined with beans, nuts and vegetables. Eat fruits alone. Apples and apple juice are the exceptions for cross-combining fruits. You can eat/drink apples with anything except animal products.

7) Timing

What and how much you eat, and how active you are from week to week are three primary factors in losing the pounds… but the fourth crucial factor is what time you eat. For starters, you might choose not to eat in the morning. This is a mistake. A latté is not breakfast. If you begin each morning with a substantial but easily digestible meal, your metabolism is jumpstarted and will continue to burn fuel throughout the day.

Another common choice is to choose one oversized meal at lunchtime. This choice causes the body to be consumed with digestion for the rest of the day, resulting in flat or negative energy. Try making time to eat simple small meals throughout the day following your morning meal (every 3-4) hours, so that by 7pm, only a small meal is needed to appease your appetite.

Most schedules dictate that dinner should be the smallest and lightest meal of the day, especially if you are not burning any energy after dinner. The last meal should generally be eaten by 7 pm. If you do have to eat later than 7p, select meals high in raw foods that are easy to digest and foods low in carbohydrates.

8) Water – Pure and filtered

Ideally you should drink about half of your body weight in ounces. This helps to rebalance the body, creating the right environment for health, cleansing, and the elimination of acidic fat cells.

Tip: Try adding lemon juice to your water to aid digestion and pull bad fats from your body. Try drinking lemon water ½ hour before meals.

9) A Daily Super-food Drink
- Having a daily green drink is essential to nourish, heal, cleanse, and energize the body. This drink should include most of the following: kelp, spirulina, chlorophyll, chlorella, wheat grass, barley grass, oat grass, apple pectin (fiber), flax seed meal, raw hemp seed protein, antioxidant rich berries (red super-foods) and other ground up vegetables.
- Try having multiple green drinks as meal replacements to expedite weight reduction.

10) 50-70% Raw Foods & Beverages
- Add powdered Matcha Green Tea to your morning super-food drink for extra energy, cleansing, anti-oxidants and a boost to your metabolism.
- Try drinking Kombucha Tea and green super-food drinks daily
- Fresh and raw vegetable juice is a great way to fill up on large quantities of nutrients.
- Eat lots of leafy greens, sprouts, broccoli, cauliflower, asparagus, carrots, celery, tomatoes, spinach, and bitter greens (kale, collards, chard).
- Try to eat two large salads daily, full of various raw veggies and a light/raw dressing.
- Grapefruit, lemons, apples, papaya and berries great fruits that aid in losing weight.
- Raw Sprouted grains: Try soaking buckwheat and steel cut oats in water over night and eat raw the next morning with nut milk and agave and cinnamon. You can find many brands at the health stores who sell raw, sprouted and dehydrated crackers, cookies, bars, bread, etc. These carbs cannot make you gain unhealthy weight! They do just the opposite.

11) Remove from Diet
- Alcohol
- Sugar-laden drinks such as soda, pasteurized fruit juice, and most sport drinks which are generally loaded with preservatives and sugar.
- Refined sugar; white flour, including bread or pasta; white rice
- Red meat that is not organic and high fat
- Processed and hydrogenated oil, canola oil, safflower oil, palm oil, vegetable oil, and/or fried foods including these oils
- Pasteurized dairy products made from cow's milk, especially milk, cream, butter and hard cheese
- Food additives and preservatives such as 'Artificial and Natural Flavors'
- Refined 'table' salt – choose 'sea salt' only
- Anything made with High Fructose Corn Syrup – the body stores this quicker as fat

12) Sprouted Cooked Grains/Carbohydrates
- The ideal way to eat cooked grains is when they have been sprouted first. The sprouting of the grain predigests the starch, increases the protein and nutrients and makes it easily digested. When cooking grains at home such as brown rice or quinoa, make sure to soak them in water over night before cooking. At health stores there are numerous varieties of already sprouted and baked products such as Ezekiel sprouted bread, pasta, tortillas, etc.

- These carbohydrates, especially brown rice, quinoa, millet, buckwheat, spelt, & amaranth, are a good source of protein and fiber to aid in cleansing the body of stored toxins and accumulated fats.
- Also include cooked fibrous complex carbohydrates such as sprouted yams, and squashes.

13) Eat Meat with Caution

If you choose to eat meat, choose the lowest mercury fish, but definitely research the origin of the fish. See Chapter 11 for guidance on seafood. Other optimal choices are eggs, turkey and chicken. Eat meat once a day, during the day or an early dinner. Try not to combine it with grains and starches – meat is easier to digest if combined only with vegetables. Choose organic, free range, grass fed meats free of hormones. Do your research on the meat source to confirm whether the meat is legitimately organic.

14) Legumes (beans)

Legumes are a good source of protein and fiber. The lightest and most nutritious are lentils (which are among the easiest to digest), soybeans, tempeh, chickpeas, white beans, and adzuki beans.

15) Good Fats, Oils and Fiber

Your body does need "good" fats in the form of Omega Fatty Acids. They can be found in raw nuts, seeds and avocados. Flaxseed oil or meal, hempseed oil and coconut oil are good fats that can actually help to pull out the bad fats, make you feel full, and aid in digestion and elimination. These oils and fibers are great additions to cleansing and sources of fiber and energy

For your daily oils, include:
1 Tbsp of raw, cold-pressed oil such as flaxseed, coconut and/or hempseed Oil. Olive oil is fine to use in moderation, as long as it is not heated.

For Omega based fibers, include:
1-2 Tbsp of ground chia seeds and/or 1-2 grams of flax seed meal and/or hempseed protein powder (ground up hemp)

I have included a sample 5+1 eating schedule on the next page for a typical all natural, high energy daily diet that will taste amazing, give you excellent energy while helping to lose weight and sustain weight loss. This is just one mix, but can easily be shuffled with other selections using the lessons and recipes in the first and second halves of this guide.

The key to changing and sustaining is keeping it new and fresh. This practice is for a lifetime so your choices will continue to evolve as you learn. Isn't that what life in general is all about? Check out the recipes at my website www.justgoodenergy.com, and use them to explore the combinations right for your energy.

AND REMEMBER - *EXERCISE!*

SAMPLE 5+1 EATING SCHEDULE FOR WEIGHT LOSS

Early morning
- ❖ A glass of water – add fresh squeezed lemon juice to aid in cleansing.
- ❖ Green drink (one serving of Amazing, Green Magma Plus, etc.) mixed with 4-8 oz. of coconut water, water, coconut milk, hemp milk and/or almond milk.)

Mid-to-late morning
- ❖ Wait at least 15-30 minutes after the green drink and have some vegetable juice (if available)
- ❖ Depending on how much energy you need, here are some suggestions: Gluten-free whole grain cereal (Chia Goodness is yum) with coconut or almond milk OR whole grain sprouted bread with a Tbsp of nut butter or coconut oil OR 1/3 cup of organic egg whites with vegetables in coconut oil and seasonings OR soaked almonds and fruit or natural yogurt, etc.

Lunch *(samples)*
- ❖ Cooked Quinoa mixed with coconut oil, Celtic Salt & nutritional yeast and crumbled tempeh over a vegetable salad
- ❖ Asian Salad – no dairy
- ❖ Salad Wrap made with "Almond Pate", avocado, veggies, goat cheese in an Ezekiel brand sprouted tortilla.

Snack
- ❖ Try having a second green drink or Young Thai Coconut, which will give your body the nutrients and satisfaction of a larger and heavier meal OR
- ❖ A couple whole grain crackers dipped in humus or raw and dairy free dip or a raw cookie/bar

Dinner (Should be concluded by 7 p.m. to 7:30 p.m.)
- ❖ If you find that your digestive tract is rejecting carbohydrates at night, I suggest having some lean protein such as tempeh, nut pates, fish, chicken or turkey with vegetables OR
- ❖ A sprouted pita, with vegetables, goat cheese and vinaigrette OR
- ❖ Non-dairy soup is also great with grilled fish OR butternut squash with olive oil and Celtic Sea Salt

Late Night Snack
- ❖ Have a Young Thai Coconut, piece of citrus fruit, papaya, kiwi, or apple

Daily Digestion:
- ❖ Have 4 oz. of Kombucha Tea ½ hour before each feeding.
- ❖ And/or take 1-2 enzymes before each breakfast, lunch and dinner.

CHAPTER
FIFTEEN

Nutrition for Mom and Baby

<u>Prenatal Care</u>

The health of your children begins in the womb. Therefore, pregnancy is the time for creating the foundation for a baby's life. Many pregnant women might mistakenly think that because they are eating for two, they can eat anything they desire and that normal rules do not apply. This is understandable. I know from experience that pregnancy is the most challenging experience we face and tests every aspect of our will and resolve as women and as humans. We are after all not robots. Our hormones are playing full court basketball like the game is on the line with every possession, and we just want peace. Food often becomes that peace, which could compromise the health of your baby.

There is a fundamental rule that we must remember when pregnant. The developing fetus only needs a mere 300-400 calories per day on average. That is the equivalent of one extra small meal, such as a bran muffin and fruit or a whole grain peanut butter and jelly sandwich and a cup of granola.

When I found out I was pregnant, I became even more aware and cautious about everything that went into my body. Even as a nutritionist, I had to acknowledge every day that I was creating a new life that is growing and evolving based on my choices, minute by minute, day by day. When you sit down to eat, ask yourself if the food is going to create healthy baby cells and tissue, or is it simply empty and nutrition-less calories that have zero positive affect. For example, if you are craving something sweet, it doesn't mean that the baby needs an ice cream sundae. Instead, revert to those rules you learned in the preceding chapters. Those same rules apply, but are even more important when you have a life growing inside you.

Below are my top 12 nutrition tips for pregnant women, which I followed my entire pregnancy all with the goal of keeping myself in optimal health and get my baby started on the right track:

1. **Choose foods closest to their natural state.** Processed and refined white flour, sugar, chips, cookies, fast food, microwave dinners, and fried foods are examples of foods which do not occur in their natural state and should be avoided or minimized. Foods in their natural state include fresh fruits and vegetables, whole grains, raw nuts and seeds, legumes, and organic meats and dairy. My personal goal is to consume a minimum of 80-90% of my daily intake from the above mentioned fresh, unaltered whole foods, especially including lots of vegetables!

2. **Baby Shake plus five.** I have found that the best way to keep up my energy, prevent heart burn, and meet the nutritional daily requirements is to eat something every 2-3 hours, beginning with a shake in the morning. It generally nets out to 1 shake plus 5 more meals. My baby shake consists of juice or water with green super-foods (Vitamineral Greens and Green Magma were my favorite), Catie's Vitamin C, protein powder, fish oil or algae DHA, yogurt and flaxseed meal. That starts me off with concentrated nutrients, healthy fats, and fiber. Then, throughout the day, don't starve yourself and the baby – eat little bits often.

3. **3 Servings of Protein Daily.** Good quality protein is essential to your baby's development and to your energy. Each serving should ideally be about 15-25 grams of protein. This doesn't mean order extra pepperoni and bacon on your pizza to meet your needs! Focus on baked or broiled organic meats and wild seafood; organic dairy; organic eggs, tempeh and miso, legumes, whole grains, nuts and seeds (chia, flax & hemp seeds). One serving of protein includes 4 ounces of meat or seafood, 3 eggs, 2 cups yogurt, or 1 cup cottage cheese. A half serving of protein includes 3 Tbsp peanut butter, 3 ounces tempeh, ¾ cup cooked beans, ½ cup of quinoa, 4 slices whole grain bread, 3 ounces nuts, ½ cup flaxseed and 2 ounces sesame seeds. Be creative and vary your proteins daily.

4. **3-4 Servings of Calcium Rich Foods Daily.** Not only does the baby need calcium to grow, it is also vital for the heart, muscle, nerve development and enzymes. Absorbable calcium is present not only in dairy, but also in vegetables, and protein-rich foods. Keep in mind that goat's milk is easier to digest than cow's milk and the calcium is much easier to assimilate. I know that you could pop a calcium pill that would give you the needed 1200 mg of required calcium, but it wouldn't be absorbed as completely or easily as whole foods. For your reference, 1 serving of about 300 mg of calcium could include 1 cup yogurt, 2 Tbsp chia seeds (5x the amount of milk), 3 tbsp sesame seeds, 1 cup cooked greens, 1½ cups edamame, 5 ounces milk, and 1 ounce cheese. If you are going to supplement, I would recommend Hydrilla Algae, which is extremely high in calcium.

5. **2 or more Servings of Iron Rich Foods Daily.** During pregnancy, your iron needs along with the baby's, are very high. It is very common for the mother to be low in iron or even anemic, which is why iron-rich foods are essential. You will know when you are even slightly low in iron because your energy will be very low, you may feel dizzy and lethargic. Good sources of iron include blackstrap molasses, seaweed, chia seeds, red meat, leafy greens (kale, collards, spinach), pumpkin seeds, tofu and tempeh, dried fruit, green grasses (wheat grass, algae spirulina) and various seafood. When supplementing iron, look for whole food based products, which are easily absorbed and do not cause constipation, such as Blood Builder by Megafoods.

6. **Half your body weight in ounces (minimum) of water daily.** Don't forget that you are also drinking for two! You and your baby are about 70% fluids and as the baby grows, so does your need for water. Drinking good quality filtered water before, during and after pregnancy helps to secure the health of mom and baby.

7. **A Good absorbable Prenatal Vitamin.** It is difficult to fulfill every needed nutrient on a daily basis. Doctors always recommend taking a prenatal. However, be cautious because not all supplements are created alike. Rather than automatically taking a prescription prenatal or a generic one from your local supermarket, do a little research first. The best prenatal to take is one that is whole food based rather than one that is made of synthetic, hard to absorb vitamins. Food based supplements digest very easily and are quickly utilized by the body. I have had great success with the Catie's Woman's Multi, New Chapter's Prenatal, and Megafoods Prenatal, all of which are food based. Also, try other products from food based brands like their calcium, iron and vitamin C.

8. **Healthy Fats and DHA.** I recommend a minimum of 3-4 servings of unrefined, raw fats on a daily average. Good fats are essential to hormone functioning, a developing baby, as well as brain and eye development (specifically needed is DHA found in fish, algae and walnuts). Try not to heat your fats whenever possible. Heated oils can change molecularly, sometimes becoming harmful, and can lose essential nutrients. Good fat sources, equivalent to about 1 serving include 1 Tbsp olive, coconut, or grapeseed oil, or 1 Tbsp chia seeds, or 2 Tbsp peanut butter, or ¼ of an avocado, or 1 tsp algal DHA or cold-pressed fish oil (rich in DHA),or 1 tsp flaxseed oil, or 3 ounces raw nuts or seeds, or 4 oz. wild salmon, or 1 Tbsp tahini.

9. **Avoid alcohol, caffeine, smoking, and drugs.** Obviously, it is dangerous to smoke or take drugs, even pharmaceutical drugs (unless approved by your doctor). The habit should ideally be eliminated cold turkey once you find out you are pregnant. Additionally, alcohol has been connected with numerous health problems in the offspring and should be avoided. Alcohol is very acidic and creates stress within your own and your baby's body. Caffeine should be minimized or avoided. If caffeine can increase your heart rate, think of what it does to the little growing baby. Also, caffeine and alcohol can prevent proper absorption of iron and calcium within the mom and baby.

10. **Minimize sodium, processed sugar and processed oils.** Read labels and make sure you are choosing low sodium foods that don't have added sugar/corn syrup or processed oils such as canola, hydrogenated oil, or fractionated palm kern oil. All three common additives are toxic, have absolutely no health benefits, cause excess weight gain for the mom and are extremely hard for the baby's body to deal with. The acid created by those chemicals is the foreground for illness, disease and other misfortunes.

11. **Eat organic whenever possible.** Organic produce, nuts and seeds, grains, etc., are as close as possible to being free of the pesticides and chemicals used in conventional foods. The fewer chemicals that you ingest, the fewer poisons that will absorb into your baby.

12. **Read labels carefully.** Words that you cannot pronounce or ingredients that are not actual foods or spices should be avoided. Here are ingredients that should raise a red flag: artificial colorings, natural flavoring, food dyes (red & yellow number 5, etc.), unnatural food additives, chemical preservatives, aspartame, MSG, sulfites, sulfur dioxide, parabens, and the list goes on. Follow the same rules you've already learned—if it is not natural, your body cannot correctly absorb and eliminate it.

Pregnancy and Baby Health: Babies are becoming increasingly acidic at birth. An acidic baby is more likely to be born preterm; have a greater chance of being overweight as a child; likely to develop diabetes and become glucose-intolerant; and are much more prone to illness. Most mothers are acidic during pregnancy. It has become much more common to become diabetic, have high blood pressure, and have a variety of stress and diet related issues. This acidic stress in the body filters to the baby.

Now it makes sense why eclampsia has become more common, which is associated with stressed and overloaded kidneys due to an abundance of waste materials (which are acidic) in the blood. If the mom consumes more alkaline foods in her diet and filtered clean water, the kidneys do not have to work as hard. At the ISIS Holistic Center, they found that, "The stress to the liver will also be reduced. This can help to prevent jaundice... Even the loss of teeth during pregnancy is common when the body is trying to obtain more alkaline minerals such as calcium".

Anemia and Pregnancy

When I was 3 months pregnant I found out that I was iron deficient, or anemic. For women, hemoglobin, (the iron-containing protein in our red blood cells) levels of less than 12 is considered anemic, while it is less than 13 for men. Iron-deficiency-anemia is not only very common amongst pregnant women, but also amongst women in general. Whether it is a result of pregnancy, blood loss during menstruation, or a lack of iron-rich foods in the diet, anemia is serious.

I could tell I was anemic without the blood tests, simply because my energy was low. I felt dizzy and was frequently short of breath. I told my doctor that rather than taking my desired prescription of 150 milligrams of iron daily, I would try to raise my iron holistically. Although meat is high in iron, it also can be difficult to digest and can be too acidic for my system. My goal was to concentrate on the easily absorbed, iron-rich foods and corresponding food-based supplements.

The result was that in four weeks, I raised my iron levels to normal. The doctor and I were both amazed at how quickly it turned around. Here is how I did it...

- I made a morning baby shake consisting of Catie's Vitamin C, Vita Mineral Green Super-foods, algal DHA, 1 Tbsp ground chia seeds, Blue-Green Algae, and Goat Milk Protein Powder—Extremely high in minerals, iron, B's, omegas, amino acids and antioxidants. I highly recommend a morning drink to everyone, not just pregnant women.
- I ate one large salad daily, consisting of a mixture of greens (spinach, arugula, dark leafy greens and sprouts) and lots of chopped red and orange vegetables. The vitamin C in vegetables and fruits (especially red and yellow ones) helped to absorb the iron in food.
- I sautéed or steamed greens such as spinach, kale, chard or other greens daily.
- I ate salmon once a week with lemon juice.
- I took 2 Tbsp of Black Strap Molasses every day with lemon juice. It sounds odd, but molasses is one of the highest food sources of iron and easier to absorb than meat.
- I avoided all caffeine and tea because the caffeine and tannins in coffee or tea can actually block absorption of iron and also calcium.
- I always separated my calcium and iron supplements and foods because when consumed together, they actually counteract each other's absorption.
- Lastly, but most importantly, I found an amazing whole food iron supplement called "Blood Builder", by Megafoods. Most iron supplements, or ferrous sulfate, are made from hard minerals like rock and steel. It is very difficult to absorb and causes much constipation! Megafoods' iron product is made from hydrilla algae, alfalfa, beet root and various other greens and algae extractions. Iron taken from natural foods, is easily recognized and utilized by the body. Each tablet contains 26 mg of Iron and all I took was 1-2 tablets daily with other greens or fruit.

Setting the Right Course for Baby

It is an age old understanding that the future health of our children is dependent upon what we as parents provide them from the time they are born. Unfortunately, this basic principle is often forgotten in the busy and increasingly artificial lifestyles that are commonplace in most circles. There are some that say, that which is free has no value, but that statement runs empty when we talk of the love we have for our children. Love is free, and is by far the most valuable gift we as parents provide our kids from the first breath. Love for our children is encased in the care we give them, and there is no more important aspect of that care than what we feed them. I believe that if you want to provide the best care for your child, then you would want to raise them on a more natural diet that is by design a more organic approach.

The first choice a mother has to make is regarding milk—breast or formula. Breast milk is the most perfect food for a baby. However, there are times when breast milk may not be available.

Goat Milk for Babies

I decided it would be smart to have an alternative to breast milk for emergencies, if my husband was watching him, or if I wasn't able to pump enough milk. I began to research the healthiest alternative to breast milk.

Goat's milk is one of the closest substances to mother's milk, next to young coconut water--very similar in vitamin and mineral ratios, digestibility, and nutrients. Goat's milk is actually the easiest milk to digest compared to every other type of milk including cow, sheep and soy. There is a lesser volume of fat molecules, and the molecules themselves are smaller. A baby's digestive system is extremely sensitive so the smaller the fat molecules, the easier it is on the baby's stomach, causing less gas and bloating. Additionally, the lactose content in goat's milk, (the protein that most people are allergic to), is very minimal compared to cow's milk.

By comparison, I know that cow's milk, in all its various forms is extremely difficult to digest. The fat molecules are very large and difficult to break down; is high in lactose and the ratio of vitamins and minerals in cow's milk are opposite to what the body needs or can break down. The only way that cow's milk is digestible is in its raw form. If you must use cow's milk only use the raw unpasteurized brands.

I also know that soy milk should have never been recommended in the first place as a formula base. It is difficult for adults to digest, provides too many estrogens, and is hard on various organs, especially the filtering organs: liver and kidneys. So just imagine how difficult a substance, soy, is for babies to digest.

It is important to note that mother's milk provides less than 2 grams of protein where goat's milk has about 7 grams per serving. A baby's system does not need that much protein, so you don't want to give them full strength, which could create too much acid in their system. So it is important to dilute the milk for easy digestibility. Goat milk should be diluted with 30-50% water.

Goat yogurt is the optimal food for the base of a formula for babies under 8 months. The culturing of goat milk into yogurt breaks down the lactose and predigests the nutrients making it very easy to assimilate. This is especially true for colicky babies. Goat yogurt formula would help their digestive tract and take very little work to digest, and will add extra probiotics for your babies' tummy health as an added plus.

Coconut Water for Babies

Young Thai Coconut water got me through my 1st trimester of pregnancy because it helped assuage my nausea and kept me hydrated. Coconut water is a nutrient-rich food high in B vitamins, alkaline minerals (electrolytes), and enzymes. In most Asian cultures, coconut water is the first liquid, besides breast milk, that is given to babies for the nutrients and the meat is pureed and offered as the baby's first food – easiest to digest.

Coconut water facts…

- More nutritious than whole cow's milk and the minerals are much more easily absorbed.
- Beneficial to pregnant women: Helps alleviate nausea, vomiting, mild laxative for common pregnancy constipation, and very nutritious.
- Beneficial to nursing moms: Creates healthy lactation.

- Coconut water is the only other food besides breast milk that contains lauric Acid – the main fatty acid in breast milk. Therefore coconut water is much healthier than processed formula from a can.

So, how can you make your own goat & coconut water formula at home for a 6 month old?

- In a bottle mix: 2 ounces of plain organic goat yogurt or milk; 2 ounces coconut water; 1 ounce of water
- Add a squirt of yacon syrup or a few drops of stevia for sweetening.
- Shake it well until the yogurt mixes with the water
  Note: If you are able to pump some breast milk, it is optimal to substitute the 1 oz of water with your breast milk.

That is all there is to it!

Again, it is important to understand that mother's milk is truly the best and is nature's perfect food for your baby. The function of this alternative formula is only an incremental supplement to mother's milk. If you were to schedule it as the primary source of food for your baby, you would have to add omegas, vitamins B12 and B6, folic acid and iron to mirror breast milk more closely.

Ready for Solids

The next phase in a baby's life is introducing solids, which can be a bit confusing and controversial. What is most interesting here is that your baby actually already has the answers for you. Babies are after all born with an innate ability to know what their bodies need and don't need. If they do eat something they perceive as foreign and unnatural, they will spit it up and most likely refuse it the next time.

Many children who contract diseases are malnourished on some level. As before mentioned, malnourished need not be always defined as starved. Quantity and quality are mutually exclusive. A child that is obese can still be malnourished because they are consuming foods lacking any nutritional value. Therefore, their bodies are lacking in vital nutrients. Poor nutrition lowers children's resistance to all kinds of diseases. It is at this young stage that malnutrition has the most severe effects; especially related to protein, iron, iodine and vitamin A deficiency.

What we can do as parents is to be smart and informed with our food selections. Ideally you would stick to as natural as possible – the less processed the better. Jarred/boxed baby food is convenient, but I challenge myself to make homemade baby food the majority of the time. Feeding your baby a variety of organic, fresh and seasonal foods is the best option and your baby will appreciate it. Any time I try to feed my son jarred foods or boxed cereals that I define as alternative, he doesn't seem to like the food as much compared to the fresh and natural course.

I'm not advising you to spend hours in the kitchen preparing meals for your baby on a daily bases. I usually make enough of each item to last 2-3 days. Another great tip I learned from another mom is to make large batches of each fruit or vegetable at a time; keep out enough for a few days and then label and freeze the rest. Next time you want to serve your baby that particular food, simply take out a portion, let it defrost in the fridge, and you are ready to serve.

Here are helpful tips I have put together for babies 6 months and older…

CEREALS:
There are two different ways to make whole grain cereal. If your baby does not have any teeth and needs to have a pureed cereal, here is what you do:
- ❖ Select from a variety of nutritious grains such as millet, amaranth, quinoa, barley, oat or rice. In a high power blender grind the grain as fine as possible.
- ❖ In a sauce pan, add about ¼ cup of the grain to just over ½ cup water (about a 1:2 ratio). Bring to a boil, reduce heat and simmer until done.

*Make sure to stir constantly or else the grain will clump. In a bowl, mix the cereal with breast milk or water if needed for thinning. Also try mixing in pureed raw fruits, mashed bananas, pureed young coconut meat, and/or a drop of raw cold-pressed coconut oil or flaxseed oil. Try different combinations of choice, depending on what they like, such as applesauce, pureed apricots, pears or mango.

FRUITS:
Try fruits that are in season. Most fruits are best when raw, unless they are really fibrous such as apples. It is difficult to puree apples completely unless precooked. Make sure and first peal any fruits that you use. Good ones to start with are peaches, apples in the form of applesauce, pears, bananas, avocado, apricots and mangos.
- • Peal the fruit, cut it into pieces, and place in your food processor or you can use a baby mill grinder.
- • Puree until smooth – add water if necessary.

VEGETABLES:
Veggies are always best when in season. Babies have a hard time digesting raw veggies, so it is always best to cook them first. Some great veggies to start your baby off with include sweet potatoes, squash, yams, green beans, peas, zucchini and carrots. I like to mix one of the orange or yellow veggies (squash, sweet potatoes, yams or carrots) with a green veggie. It makes it a bit more palatable. However, some babies like peas or green beans by themselves, try and see what happens.

PROTEIN:
Generally between 9-12 months, babies are ready for a small amount of protein-rich foods. Depending on your baby, you could introduce animal protein such as chicken, fish, goat cheese, legumes, and eggs. Legumes such as lentils, white beans, adzuki and black beans should only be given if they are first soaked in water for 18-24 hours before cooking. The soaking process allows pre-digestion to begin, breaks down the enzyme inhibitors in the bean, and increases the absorbability of the protein and nutrients. As a result, the body has less digestive lag time (no gas or bloating).

COMBINATION MEALS:
Once a baby is used to the individual grains, veggies and proteins, it is really fun to begin making pureed soups and stews. My son loves when I cook together sprouted quinoa, soaked red lentils, chopped carrots, and acorn squash. I simply placed all ingredients in a pot with some water, bring to a boil, cool, and then puree. I like to add a little coconut oil, Celtic Sea salt and nutritional yeast. I make enough for at least 10 meals, freezing enough for 3 meals per container.

Another fun recipe is cauliflower mashed potatoes. I steam the cauliflower and butternut squash until really soft and then puree with olive oil, Celtic sea salt, nutritional yeast and coconut water. YUM! Be creative.

LIQUIDS:
After 6 months it is recommended to start offering your baby fluids besides breast milk or formula. Rather than give my son juice, which is full of sugar, I like to offer him water, a little bit of diluted goat milk, or a few ounces of Young Coconut water (not to be confused with coconut milk). The coconut water is great on their tummies and aids in digestion. It is refreshing for them while not too filling. I buy a couple of the Young Coconuts from the health food store weekly, chop it open, drain out the water, and use over 2-3 days. You can also freeze the coconut water and use at a later time.

FATS:
Breast milk and formula have all the fat needed for an infant. However, as your baby starts nursing less and eating more solids, gradually they will need some fat to be added to their solid regime. One of the best fats is avocado – great pureed with banana, applesauce, sweet potatoes, or by itself. The oils that I commonly add are coconut oil, flaxseed oil and olive oil. Plain goat yogurt is also an easily digested fat/protein/calcium. My son absolutely loves pureed peaches with unsweetened goat yogurt. Sometimes I add a couple drops of yacon Syrup or stevia. It is also great as a kefir type drink. Combine part goat yogurt with water, breast milk or coconut water and shake well.

MORE TIPS:
- I don't recommend adding salt to any of your baby's food until they are at least 9 months. If you are going to add salt, add minimally and the only salt that should be used is Celtic Sea Salt or Himalaya Salt, which are whole foods supplying over 80 minerals. Since a baby's kidneys can't handle a large amount of sodium, it is best to eliminate all processed salts.
- Try not to sweeten any foods as much as possible. Even with plain goat yogurt, first let them taste it plain before adding anything sweet to it. If you are going to use any sweetener, it is best to stick to fresh fruits, agave, maple syrup, barley malt, rice syrup or stevia, making sure to avoid honey until after one year.
- Try rotating foods every 3-4 days to insure that your baby is getting a varied diet.
- Wait 3 to 4 days before introducing a new food.
- Don't force-feed your baby, they know what they need.
- Always buy organic whenever possible.

FUNCTIONAL FOODS FOR KIDS

Food plays such an integral part of our daily lives, especially for kids and teens. Like their parents, kids are moving through their days faster than ever, switching gears hourly as they maneuver through their obstacle course like schedules, all the while expected to think, respond, and perform with maximum mental clarity. Their day doesn't end with the last class, but most often continues with little rest as they must be on time for their after school sports practice, or the countless array of extra-curricular activities.

What use is going to class if one is too tired and hungry to digest the information their teachers are feeding them. I remember so many classes, even in college, where I was sitting in my desk, but was not quite present. Our expectations for our kids to perform at the highest level are naturally high, but a sprouting child or hormone fluctuating teen can't take all the blame for falling asleep in class, being late, or just losing focus altogether if we are not giving them the tools to create natural, sustained energy that can keep them going all day. The energy you help them create as they are growing will be a feeling they will not forget, and they may not feel the pressure to improve their performance through synthetic means. How our kids fuel can absolutely make the difference in how well they are building their foundation and ultimately how they experience their daily schedule. This schedule graduates week after week, month-to-month, and each year, becoming more complex. Ideally, you can help them establish a life-long foundation for learning, discovering, experiencing and becoming. Of course, we must all lead our children by example so the lifestyle must start with us, and filter into them. Inconsistencies between our actions and their actions will lead to inconsistencies in their behavior.

The most available and non-synthetic tool available to create a strong foundation is food. Functional foods are the key--not empty calories, sugars, and fast food. Functional means the ability to serve a purpose for which it was designed; therefore, functional foods have been designed to promote mental clarity and focus, physical and mental energy, emotional balance and overall development. Such foods include whole grains, raw and unprocessed fats, vegetables, nuts, seeds, lean white meat, fish, fruit, and legumes. Eating for kids should be a fun experience and it is the best time to introduce new foods, while they are developing their tastes. Kids need to picture healthy, functional foods the same way they see a new pair of sneakers for basketball. That new pair of shoes will ignite them to run faster and jump higher, just as that pita sandwich with veggies will make them think and focus quicker and longer, and will prevent the radical ups and downs that excess sugars cause. No difference really, just a paradigm shift in how your child perceives foods. If you start from day one, than their need not be a shift. Their perception of foods will be as it should be.

My view is that healthy foods in their natural state can be more interesting and fun for your kids. The key is to induce passion for understanding foods and how they affect your body and mind so that the word, "yuck!" is their response when they see a fried burger, fries, and soda. Imagine that! Help them understand that dead, lifeless, overly processed food is yuck because it actually depletes their energy. Lead and they will follow.

I've included snack ideas below that you can teach your kids to make. These foods are functional in the sense that they provide optimal energy and give them the nutrition they need on many levels as they glide through their daily transitions…

Kid-Friendly High-Energy Snacks
- ☺ Triangle quesadillas (whole grain tortilla with goat cheddar or rice cheese)
- ☺ Tortilla roll sandwich (Spread over a whole grain tortilla, some Veganaise or humus, sandwich toppings, veggies, etc and then roll it up and cut in half
- ☺ Homemade veggie burrito
- ☺ Scrambled eggs in a whole grain pita half
- ☺ Mini homemade Pizza on whole English muffin or bread with favorite toppings, toasted
- ☺ Frozen grapes are a great sweet treat
- ☺ Peanut butter and banana sandwich (try Alvarado sprouted bread or whole grain bread)
- ☺ Pureed yams in a cup (bake a yam and then puree it with a little salt and honey – yum)
- ☺ Homemade chicken strips (leftovers from last night's dinner)

☺ Yam fries (bake 1 or more yams for 25 minutes at 425 degrees, peel, cut in ½ lengthwise, and then cut 1 inch strips, lay them on a baking sheet greased with grapeseed or coconut oil, sprinkle a little sea salt on the fries and then bake for about 15 minutes on each side at 425 degrees. Delicious!

☺ Fruit sweetened yogurt

☺ Whole grain crackers (Kashi, Dr. Cracker, Flat Bread crackers, etc.)

☺ Natural, fruit sweetened granola in a baggy (try Nature's Path, Kashi, Ezekiel, Go Raw, ...)

☺ Smoothie and juice

☺ Smoothies made with Amazing Grass Kidz Super-foods, frozen fruit, almond milk and yogurt

☺ Frozen juice is a great replacement for popsicles

☺ Raw almonds, walnuts or peanuts with raisins

☺ Chopped raw veggies

CHAPTER
SIXTEEN

Supplement/Product Recommendations

My greatest emphasis is on "Whole Food Supplementation". This means that nutrients are added to the diet through whole and natural food sources rather than synthetic and extracted vitamins or minerals. Taking individual vitamins, minerals, antioxidants, etc., are not meant to be a replacement for eating healthy foods or a band-aid for eating an unhealthy diet. Get as much variety and nutrients through whole foods and then supplement as naturally and wholesomely as possible, being careful not to overdo it! I personally take red and green super-foods and sea vegetables daily in place of a general multivitamin, along with eating very balanced. Below is a list of my most recommended whole food supplements.

Green Super-food Blend
One scoop daily on an empty stomach (mixed in water or juice). I personally take the greens daily instead of taking a multivitamin, along with eating very balanced. These blends should include a variety of green grasses and sea vegetables, such as wheat grass, spirulina, chlorophyll, barley grass, hydrilla, alfalfa, kelp, etc. These are high in vitamins, minerals, aminos, proteins, omegas, and enzymes. Make sure they are dried at less than 110 degrees

> ❖ **Vitamineral Greens** www.healthforce.com
> Amazing Grass www.amazinggrass.com
> Catie's Greens www.energyessentials.com
> Dr. Tony's "Radiant Greens" www.calcompnutrition.com
> Green Magma www.greenfoods.com

Red and Purple Super-foods
"Powerful Antioxidant Super-foods" Gogi Berries (Wolf Berries), Schizandra Berries, Pomegranates, Acai Fruit, Grapes/Grapeseed, Lycopene (extract from Tomatoes) Mangosteen Plant, and Red and Purple Berries such as Blueberries, Cranberries and Bilberries. They have been proven to fight and deactivate the hundreds of pollutants and pesticides we inhale and ingest daily. The following health-promoting characteristics are shared by these powerful fruits: High in antioxidants, minerals, amino acids, trace minerals, energy, stamina, and are anti-inflammatory, alkalizing, boosts the immune system, powerhouse of nutrition, anti-aging, environmental protectors, stimulates mental function, and balances the nervous system. I recommend taking a combination of the fruits daily in a concentrated/fresh powder or juice. There are various companies coming up with amazing combinations of powder versions of all or most of these fruits combined.

> ❖ Dr. Tony's Pomegranate Power www.calcompnutrition.com/pomegranate-power.html
> Catie's Vitamin C Plus www.energyessentials.com

Blue-Green Algae

1 tsp or 4 capsules daily along with the green super food blend. It is one of the highest greens in omegas, chlorophyll, proteins, and immune building properties—also great for environmental protection, inflammation and focus.

> ❖ Ancient Sun's Crystal Manna Wild Blue-green algae (flakes) – from Klamath Lake in Oregon. They also make a powder/capsule called Blue Manna, which I highly recommend. It is much more concentrated and specifically is for brain and joint health. Take 1/3 tsp or 2 caps daily.
> (Recommended adding 1 tsp of the flakes and 1/3 tsp of the Blue Manna to your morning green food super-blend daily, and up to 3 Tbsp if you are feeling like you are getting sick or are already sick, have low energy, or are nutritionally deficient)

EPA and DHA

EPA and DHA are the noteworthy components naturally provided in algae and raw, cold-pressed fish and flaxseed oil. "Algal DHA is a healthier form of **pure DHA and Omega 3** (fish get their DHA up the food chain from algae), and it does not endanger fish populations. It also does not contain any mercury or any other contaminant found in fish. The special algae are grown in environmentally sustainable tank farms, just as they grow spirulina. Several studies have shown that algal DHA is more easily utilized by the body. Also algal DHA does not have the saturated fat content that fish oil has, so algal DHA is actually better for the heart and arteries than fish (or krill) oil." This was C Admas' comment on Algal DHA who is a Naturopath who holds a Ph.D. in Natural Health Sciences, a Doctorate of Sciences in Integrative Health, and a degree in Traditional Naturopathy, and more.

DHA is important for the brain, focus, and ADD. Algal DHA, chia seeds, fish and flax oil are also very high in Omega 3, which is important for hair, skin, cells, a balanced central nervous system, strong immune system, hormone regulation, brain function, mood control, heart health, and much more. Make sure that any oils that you take are raw/cold-pressed. I highly recommend taking 2-3 grams of algal DHA, fish and/or flaxseed oil. When taking Fish oil, make sure the oil has been tested for mercury and other metals, is from a very good source and has been molecularly distilled.

Evening Primrose Oil (EPO)

1-2 grams daily as needed. EPO comes form the seeds of the evening primrose plant. EPO contains gamma linolenic acid (GLA). EPO/GLA has been used in connection with the following conditions: diabetes, eczema, osteoporosis, PMS, arthritis (due to its anti-inflammatory properties), skin ulcers, and breast disease.

Protein Enzymes

1-3 capsules daily on an empty stomach as a maintenance. Protein enzymes, including bromelain, protease, papain, and other varieties are key to life. They aid in inflammation, re-growth, repairing, immune building, bacteria fighting and anti-aging.

> ❖ Enzymedica's "Repair", "Repair Gold" and/or "Virastop" (For an injury, illness, or body trauma, take 3, 2-3 times/day.)

Digestive Enzymes

1-3 capsules, depending on need, before meals. Aiding in digestion, assimilation, and prevention of acid, indigestion and purification.

> ❖ Enzymedica's "Digest" or "Digest Gold" www.enzymedica.com

Digestive Disorders

Aside from Acidophilus, there are various herbs that can help to heal the GI tract, digestive lining, mucous membrane health of the digestive system, and sooth the bowels. The most gentle include Okra, ginger, turmeric, chlorella regularis, Sea Buckthorn berries/oil, raw coconut oil and Calendula.

Fiber

25-35 mg daily. If you don't get enough fiber in your diet, try consuming 1-2 Tbsp of cold-pressed flaxseed meal or chia seeds. Mix it in liquids or sprinkle on un-heated food.

Acidophilus/Probiotics

The Chinese believe that the stomach is the key to our entire body's health. If you think about it, almost everything we consume is received, processed and distributed from the stomach. This is where the essential probiotics, commonly known as acidophilus, come in. Probiotics are the friendly flora, or bacteria, that support the normal colon ecology for digestion, absorption, elimination, and prevention of yeasts, bacteria and parasites. Simply put, they are the soldiers which keep our stomach, intestines and colon clean and happy.

Unfortunately, we are constantly surrounded by toxins and stresses, both internally and externally, which can wreak havoc on our bodies. The good bacteria in our GI tract is directly affected and becomes a casualty of war; good versus bad bacteria. If the stomach and intestinal area is toxic and laden with harmful bacteria, how do we expect our bodies to stay strong and healthy with a toxic life-force? With the depletion of good flora comes the harmful bacteria and yeast which can monopolize the entire digestive track. As a result the body can become very acidic and prone to illness, yeast infections, candida, digestive disorder, and much more. Also keep in mind that taking antibiotics actually kills the friendly flora in your system, making your body much more susceptible to illness.

It is recommended to take 3 or more billion live organisms of probiotics daily as maintenance. The most common forms of acidophilus found in supplemental forms include: lactobacillus acidophilus (the original strain); lactobacillus casei; lactobacillus bulgaricus; Bifidobacterium bifidum. There are a variety of others.

❖ One of the most absorbable and potent probiotics available is "Bio-K", which is a raw liquid form containing over 50 billion live cultures per serving. They make a great fermented rice-based organic product that is amazing.

Coenzyme Q10

30-60 mg. is the average daily dose for maintenance. CoQ10 is made by the body and also found in oily fish (in the EPA) and whole grains. It is a fat-soluble vitamin that is essential to the body's energy systems, is an immune stimulant, lowers the blood pressure, supports heart function, promotes healthy skin, and supports longevity. CoQ10 is best absorbed when formulated with mixed tocopherols (from Vitamin E) – it should read "Tocopherols" on the ingredient list. Look for liquid-in-a-capsule varieties and not the powdered CoQ10.

Multi Vitamin & Mineral

Low dosage liquid (preferable), capsule or tablet 5-6 days of the week. Stick to a plant/food-based, organic, all natural multiple with no fillers or preservatives. I generally recommend "multi's" for those not eating a healthy balanced diet, are low in nutrients, or don't take any of the green super food blends regularly.

❖ There are some companies which make 100% food-based and 90-100% organic supplements, such as Catie's and Mega Foods.

MSM

2-3 grams daily for inflammation, arthritis, tendonitis, collagen reproduction, skin/hair/nail health, and over-use of joints and muscles. MSM is the natural sulfur-containing nutrient found in cells, occurring widely in nature. This nutritional sulfur is a mineral vital to protein synthesis and balanced health. Sulfur is constantly being used up within the body, and depletion causes degenerative conditions. MSM is a great rebuilding nutrient and preventative.

Amino Acids

For those concerned about protein intake or not getting the full-spectrum of essential amino acids, there are some great natural sources available. Aminos made from sea vegetables is the best absorbed and friendliest to the body. Other food sources include Green Super-foods, especially Blue-Green Algae, Hydrilla, and other plant-based Amino supplements.

Calcium/Magnesium

600-1200mg is the daily recommendation. Most women don't get enough calcium and benefit well from supplementing approximately 500 mg of calcium and magnesium. The most mass produced calcium supplements are in the form of calcium carbonate, calcium citrate, MCHA calcium, and coral calcium. Those forms of calcium are either from dried rocks or animal bones, which are very difficult for the body to break down and absorb. Too much of the non-plant based calcium can cause calcification and calcium stones. Make sure the supplement is plant-based, and ideally a liquid or powder. You can get most if not all of the recommended calcium from vegetables, seeds, especially chia seeds, whole grains, green super foods, sea vegetables, beans and many other foods. Try to absorb as much of your daily calcium from foods, and supplement with plant-based calcium according to your daily demand.

Hydrilla

Hydrilla is a type of algae, as mentioned above, superior in calcium. It is also an abundant source of magnesium, manganese, potassium, zinc, copper, B vitamins, C, E, Iron, Chlorophyll Amino Acids, Fatty Acids, and essential trace minerals. This amazing algae also acts as a powerful antioxidant, scouring the body for free radicals. You can find Hydrilla in supplemental form, usually in 400-500 mg per capsule. I recommend 1-2 capsules daily.

> ❖ The optimum food source of Calcium is Hydrilla, which is a type of algae that is more absorbable and superior than any other form of supplemental/extracted calcium. Other great sources of calcium used in food-based supplements include Kelp, alfalfa, and various sea vegetables. Catie's Calcium and Mega Foods Cal/Mag are both made from mainly Hydrilla Algae, but also include other sea veggies and alfalfa.

Match Green Tea

Consuming green tea regularly is very beneficial to one's health. "Matcha" tea, specifically, is very high in antioxidants, minerals, immune building properties, and is a great source of energy, focus and mental clarity. "Matcha" Green tea is known as "Ceremonial Tea", used for optimal clarity and meditation. I recommend 1-3 tsp daily mixed with water or blended into a smoothie. It is a great replacement for coffee and other harmful caffeinated beverages.

Adding to Your Energy Pool

The question I get asked the most is, "I never have enough energy…what can I do? Your energy levels change throughout the day. Start paying attention to these energy shifts and the behaviors that might be factoring in to the shift in levels. For example, you can ask yourself, 'What did you just eat?' 'Are you stressed?' 'Has it been more than 2-3 hours since eating something?' 'Did you have sugar or caffeine prior to feeling tired?' 'Did you sleep well the night before?' 'Did you eat heavier foods the previous evening?'

So many factors can influence our energy. Did you know that food digestion takes more energy from your body than anything else? I've listed out some sources of energy on the following page that can assist you as you try to balance your energy naturally.

- Acai, Schizandra, Rhodiola, and Goji Berry - High energy & antioxidant berries.
- Maca Root - A South American superfood that is dense in nutrients such as protein and calcium, high in antioxidants, and is well known for it's ability to increase energy and endurance, along with balancing the hormones.
- Cordyceps Mushroom - Great for overall energy and immune system (this is a favorite with athletes needing that long endurance boost.
- Green Tea/Matcha Tea - Keeps the energy, stamina, focus and metabolism going
- Yerba Mate Tea - good energy boost and great replacement for coffee
- Green Super-foods - Wheat, Barley and other green grasses, Blue-Green Algae, Sea Vegetables, Spirulina, Chloryphyll, (high in Iron, minerals, Aminos, B vitamins, and natural energy)
- Eleuthero Ginseng, also known as Siberian Ginseng
- CoQ10 - Great for the heart, the brain, cellular energy, immune system, and even amazing for your gums
- Ashwaganda (Ayurvedic Herb) - An adaptogenic herb that increases the body's overall energy

Antioxidants, Immune Builders and Anti-Virals/Bacterials

There are many healing herbs and vitamins that are optimal for boosting the immune system as needed, whether you are traveling, feeling sick, surrounded by illness, or maintaining. Many of these powerful herbs protect against environmental toxins. Did you know that we ingest over 300 pounds of toxins yearly? Such toxins include pollution, pesticides, herbicides, carbon monoxide, tar, ash and many more.

- ❖ Our helpful fighters include: Mushroom complex's (Maitake, Shitake, Cordyceps), Grape Seed, Vitamin C, Quercitin, Olive Leaf, Turmeric (also for inflammation), Briar Rose, Stinging Nettle, Echinacea, Ginger, Oregano Oil, Goldenseal, Bee Propelis, Bromelain, Yerba Santa, Elderberry, Garlic, and Astragalus. These are some of my favorites and many come in combinations or singularly. They are most potent in the liquid or dried extract form! See what works best for you.

Stress and Mood Support

There are various plants and berries which can provide natural stress, anxiety, depression, and emotional relief. Not only do they lift you up, but they can balance your central nervous system while giving energy to the entire body. Some commonly used herbs are Rhodiola Berry (100-300 mg), Schizandra Berry, Holy Basil, Eleuthero, and Ashwaganda. I have known people with severe depression successfully use Rhodiola Berry to reduce and eliminate the need for pharmaceutical anti-depressants. Schizandra, Eleuthero and Ashwaganda can also help balance those with underactive adrenals and thyroid gland.

❖ **Ayurvedics & Stress Balance**

I am impressed by a product that we have been using in my family for more than a year called **StressCare by Himalaya.** It is a unique complex of Ayurvedic Herbs with strong adaptogenic actions that help cope with life's daily stress. Ayurveda is translated as the "knowledge of life". The central theory of Ayurvedic medicine is based in India and claims that health exists when there is a synergistic balance within the body. Specifically, they believe in three fundamental systems in the body known as Vata (nervous system), Pitta (digestion/metabolism) and Kapha (fluids/lubrication/arterial system).

Adaptogenic herbs work with your body to find the necessary healing and balance needed rather than forcing any actions on it. Rather than taking a single herb for stress like Ashwaganda or Rhodiola Berry, Himalaya has combined over a dozen herbs that work together synergistically to balance not only the nervous system but every other organ and system in the body. It offers a broad range of health benefits and balances all the body's organs and systems for increased mental alertness and greater physical fitness.

Many health conditions today have been connected to physical and mental stress and anxiety. It is not enough to put a band aid on stress by taking pharmaceutical drugs, therefore ignoring the real problems and needs of the body. We need balance on every level: spiritually, nutritionally, emotionally, and physically. While it is important to de-stress through relaxation, exercise, meditation and natural foods, herbs can enhance the balancing process and feed the body's systems.

Ayurvedic stress-related herbs can act as a support system to your body's needs. *Stress Care* is a completely natural product that regulates and balances all of the body's organs and systems for comprehensive health maintenance. *Stress Care* provides several vitamins and minerals from natural sources, enabling the formula to deliver a broad range of health benefits on top of stress management. It provides strong antioxidant properties, the key to its anti-aging benefits, and improves hormonal effectiveness, the key to its menopausal benefits. Other stress-related conditions which can be alleviated include premature aging, emotional imbalance, insomnia, mental alertness, and physical condition.

Prostate & Urinary Tract Supplementation

Saw Palmetto, Stinging Nettle, Pumpkin seed, Cranberry, and Pygeum bark are great herbs, which support the strengthening, and functioning of the prostate and urinary tract. Acidophilus is also important for urinary tract cleanliness and function.

Gentle Laxative

One of the most gentle and non-habit forming laxatives is Triphala. This is an Ayurvedic herb used for thousands of years for regulating the bowel system and elimination functions, along with strengthening digestion and nutritional assimilation. This herb is safe for all ages. It is recommended to take 2 capsules (almost 500 mg) before bed with water as needed. Aloe Vera, available in a capsule or as a liquid, is another mild laxative which has a soothing effect while cleansing the colon. I don't, however, recommend taking Aloe Vera daily, due to its ability to pull out some of your good minerals. Use it maybe 1-3 times per week as needed before bed. Flaxseed Meal can be used daily, about 1-2 Tbsp and is a gentle cleanser that keeps you regular. A high potent Acidophilus can also be very beneficial.

Part III

SETTING UP YOUR KITCHEN

Chapter 17
Good Energy Appliances

Chapter 18
Choosing your Foods

Chapter 19
Natural Alternative Substitutions

CHAPTER SEVENTEEN

Good Energy Appliances

When setting up your kitchen it is important to have the right tools for the right job. Below is a list of the appliances we recommend and find most helpful:

Blender / Grinder
Choose an upright heavy-duty variety with several speeds. The best one we have found is the *Vitamix Total Nutrition Center*. We use blenders when making milks, sauces, seed and nut yogurts and drinks. Grinders are used in processing grains, seeds and nuts into a flour mixture. The *Vitamix* has a dry canister that is great for grinding whole sprouted grains, seeds and nuts.

Juicer
A juice extractor plays an important role in the creation of many of our recipes. One of our favorite juicers is the Green Power. It is powered by gears instead of a motor and minimizes the heat generated in the process of extracting juices from fruits and vegetables. It can be used for making wheat grass juice. We also like the Champion juicer. Juicers are good for making nut butter, juices, pates, cookies, and frozen fruit sorbets and other desserts.

Citrus Juicer/Squeezer
We use this for making fresh lemon and lime juice -- ingredients in many of our recipes -- as well as fresh orange and grapefruit juice.

Dehydrator
We prefer the Excalibur, s*ee appendix for web address*. It has several adjustable and removable trays with a choice of using thin sheets that allow you to dehydrate thinner, more liquid mixtures. The heat blows from back to front, creating more even drying. Its adjustable, removable trays allow you to dehydrate pie shells in their pie plates and nut loaves in their casserole dishes. This is the most versatile dehydrator we have found. We dehydrate sprouted grains, herbs and spices, grain burgers, cookies, crackers, vegetables and fruit.

Food Processor
Food processors typically have a wider opening and a larger blade than a standard blender. This makes it easier to create chunkier mixtures for raw pâtés, burgers, crackers and cookies and piecrusts. It is also great for making cookie dough. A salad shooter is an inexpensive hand-held food processor that has different blade attachments for thin slicing and grating fruits, vegetables and cheeses.

Wheat Grass Juicer
You can make your own wheat grass juice with the Green Power juice extractor, an electric wheat grass juicer, or a hand wheat grass juicer.

CHAPTER
EIGHTEEN

Choosing Your Foods

Choose Organic

Your produce, grains, legumes, seeds and nuts are only as nutritious as the ground they come from, so whenever you can, buy organic. In order for a food to be labeled "organic" the soil it came from must be free of chemicals and pesticides for 10 years, and the growers must only use organic fertilizer. The organic matter used by organic growers brings fertility back to the soil, which has been neglected by conventional farmers. While the rise of pesticides and synthetic fertilizers has increased tenfold in the last forty years, crop losses due to insects have doubled. Organic methods, on the other hand, build up the soil, creating stronger, more disease-resistant plants.

Most people would be surprised to know that while 10% of the pesticides ingested in our country come from produce, 90% are found in animal products. Produce is treated with pesticides a set number of times during its growth, while factory farm animals are fed pesticide-laden crops regularly. The pesticides eaten daily by the animals are absorbed into their tissues and stored there. When you eat these animals or the milk products they produce, you are consuming concentrated doses in uncontrolled combinations of many of the most deadly chemicals ever known.

Eating organic is the only way to guarantee that you are receiving the nutrition that nature intended, while reducing the volume of toxic chemicals entering your systems. You will find that organic produce is much more flavorful. If you are home growing, buy organic seeds, fertilizer or composts. If you choose to eat processed foods, buy organic, and if you choose to eat meat, buy free range.

Cleaning Your Food

Whether you buy organic or not, you should clean your produce, grains, legumes, nuts and seeds in water. There are many cleansers on the market which will remove up to 90 percent of the pesticides and bacteria from non-organic food. The other 10 percent of the pesticides have been absorbed by the food and cannot be removed.

Checking Labels

Read labels carefully; or you won't know what you are eating. Stay away from chemical preservatives, refined sugars, oils and salts. When selecting processed foods, look for those foods which have more nutritious ingredients, and fewer additives.

Sweeteners

Refined sweeteners are unhealthy. Buy only raw, organic, unrefined sweeteners.

Below is a list of sweeteners that we use and recommend:

❖ **Featured Sweetener: Yacon Syrup**

"*Yacon* Root is a raw, low-calorie, low-sugar, molasses-like flavored syrup with a broad-spectrum nutrient profile. With special, natural fructoligosaccharide (FOS) sugars enables Yacon to be absorbed and used as a prebiotic or "food" in the digestive tract.

Great for diabetics and sugar sensitivities, dieters, healthy diets, digestive imbalances, high cholesterol, and also aiding in athletic performance; making it an incredible, natural, top notch whole food and a sweetener to boot! It has been found and studied that *Yacon* syrup has very little influence on insulin spiking and is dramatically less glycemic-effect than sugar, honey, agave and/or maple syrup.

Yacon is rich in Potassium, Phosphorus, Chromium, Calcium, Iron, Copper, and other trace minerals. It contains a whole B complex profile, important antioxidants and 11% complete protein by dry weight. Use it as you would any sweetener -- in food recipes and in beverages, teas, coffee, smoothies, etc." (Darin Olin, Darin's Naturals)

Learn more about this fantastic new sweetener at: www.darinsnaturals.com

---

Honey - Honey is a simple carbohydrate that is easily digested. It is more concentrated than white refined sugars, so use less. Honey comes from the nectar of blossoms that bees gather and convert into food. There are many different varieties and flavors, so try different ones. The darker the honey, the more minerals it has. All honey should be purchased raw and unfiltered. If it crystallizes, put the container in warm water (never boiling water), to liquefy it again. If honey is not raw, then the concentrated sugar content becomes more difficult to digest. Only raw honey contains the necessary enzymes to digest itself in your body, and it aids in the digestion of other foods eaten at the same time.

Coconut Nectar – Raw, low glycemic and nutritious sweetener made from coconut sap. Rich in minerals, B's and has a neutral PH. http://www.coconutsecret.com/nectar2.html

Maple Syrup - Maple syrup is seasonal and derived from the sap of the maple tree. There is no such thing as "raw" maple syrup because it is boiled during processing. It takes 40 gallons of sap to make one gallon of syrup. Because it is boiled, maple syrup has fewer nutrients than honey, but the flavor is unique and milder. Use only Organic Grade A 100 percent maple syrup, and avoid anything that says "maple-flavored" syrup.

Maple sugar - It is the crystallized form of maple syrup – the raw version is more of a whole food and can be a useful natural alternative to refined sugar.

Date Syrup - Date Syrup comes from soaking dates and blending them in the same water that they were soaked in.

Date Sugar - It comes from ground dehydrated dates and is really not a sugar at all, but a ground-up food. It is a great sweetener, but it does not dissolve in liquids, which can pose problems while cooking.

Brown Rice Syrup and Barley Malt Syrup - Both are complex carbohydrates that enter the digestive system slowly and don't cause an imbalance in blood-sugar levels. They are mild sweeteners with trace minerals and nutrients.

Bananas - Bananas can be used to sweeten and thicken sauces and baked foods. If frozen and put through a juice extractor, they are a wonderful replacement for frozen sorbet or ice cream.

Carrots and Onions – Both help to sweeten cooked foods.

Dried Fruit Purees - Soaked, dried fruits pureed in their own soaked water make great sweeteners. Some choices are raisins, dates, prunes, peaches and currants.

Xylitol - Xylitol is the commercial name for the natural sweetener, Xylose, derived from the Birch tree. The significant difference between xylose and most sugars is that the xylose molecule contains only 5 carbon atoms rather than the 6 of most other sugars. This molecular difference is the key to xylitol's healthful benefits. Like stevia, xylitol does not feed intestinal yeast, and does not raise insulin or blood sugar levels. This makes it a healthy sugar replacement for diabetics. It tastes like sugar, but has 40% less calories and does not create that sugar high or low. Xylitol can be mixed in hot or cold beverages or baked with, using equal amounts to sugar (i.e. 1 Cup sugar= 1 Cup xylitol). However, xylitol is not as sweet as syrups such as honey and maple, so per 1 cup of honey you would probably need about 1 1/3 cup of xylitol.

> ❖ **Stevia** - Stevia is a clear or golden liquid measured by the dropper; or white powder used by the teaspoonful. It is about 40 times sweeter than sugar and is very nutritious. It is grown in South America and is an extract from the Stevia rebaudiana leaf. Stevia has been shown to have several important health benefits associated with the regulation of blood sugar and blood pressure. It's great for diabetics. Use it in beverages and any sauces or dishes. (See replacement amounts.) This is a whole food and is better for you if it is not used in an extracted form.

Condiments

Condiments, other than herbs and spices, can enhance the flavors of other foods. Fresh condiments that most people are familiar with include garlic, onions, chives, lemon juice, ginger, chilies, bell pepper, and grated carrot.

The following list includes other less-familiar condiments that we use regularly:

Miso - Be sure to use the paste, because powdered miso is inferior in taste and almost devoid of nutrition. Miso is derived from fermented soybeans, legumes, or whole grains. It is a fermented paste that adds a lot of flavor and is high in minerals and enzymes.

> ❖ **Nama Shoyu** – The only 100% raw, unpasteurized soy sauce that is Non-GMO and can be found organic; is rich in enzymes, acidophilus and flavor, and is considered "The Champagne of Soy Sauces" Nama Shoyu is naturally aged for four years and lower in sodium. www.rawganique.com/Food1.htm

Coconut Aminos – Made from the sap of coconuts. Raw, organic, fermented, rich in 17 amino acids, blended with sun-dried mineral-rich sea salt and nutritious—a healthy and tasty alternative to traditional soy sauce or Braggs with a slightly sweeter and less salty flavor. http://www.coconutsecret.com/aminos2.html

Tamari Sauce - It is a naturally fermented soybean sauce that is wheat free and more concentrated than regular soy sauce, (which is usually made from wheat and is about 20 percent salt). Salt is added to tamari sauce, rather than being a natural ingredient. If you buy tamari sauce, use the low-sodium variety.

Raw Tahini - Tahini is a seed butter that thickens and helps to make soups, sauces and patés creamier. It has been used in the Middle East for thousands of years as a dairy substitute. It is nutritious and is an easily digested unsaturated fat. It is high in calcium, magnesium, phosphorous and protein.

Nutritional Yeast - This yeast is a golden flake that is sold in health food stores and is high in B Vitamins (especially in Vitamin B-12), folic acid, amino acids and minerals. It adds a nutty, cheese-like flavor to sauces, soups and dressings, or it can be sprinkled on top of salads. Don't confuse nutritional yeast with brewers yeast. Nutritional yeast is grown as a food and food supplement. Brewers yeast is a by-product. Choose a brand that is grown in a controlled environment (below 115 degrees) which helps to retain its raw state.

Vegetarian Chicken, Vegetable or Beef Broth - This product is a combination of whole grain flour, dehydrated vegetables, potato flour, spices, and herbs. It helps flavor soups, gravies, and sauces. Check the labels for additives and MSG before buying.

Psyllium - Psyllium is made from plantago seed husks. We use it in small amounts as a thickener in raw desserts and some sauces.

Sauerkraut (raw) - Sauerkraut is a sliced and naturally fermented cabbage. It provides beneficial enzymes and friendly bacteria and aids in digestion.

Vinegars - Buy organic; brown rice, apple cider, red wine, and Balsamic or UME Boshi Plum vinegar. The UME vinegar is a salty Japanese vinegar made from Japanese vegetables. It has a pickled flavor, and is a high alkaline food allowing for easier digestion.

Worcestershire Sauce - Buy the natural version with no MSG, preservatives or added salt. Robbies is a great brand.

Barbecue Sauce - Robbies brand is all natural.

Mustard - Traditional yellow mustard is difficult to digest and is hard on your colon. The Dijon varieties are better. If you choose to use either, read the ingredients.

Catsup - Buy organic versions that are fruit or honey sweetened: common catsup is usually very high in sugar and sodium. Non-organic tomato sauces and catsup are not properly regulated, so companies frequently use over-ripened tomatoes containing insects and other undesirables.

Mayonnaise - If you choose to use mayonnaise, use eggless and dairy free.

> ❖ The natural alternative product we recommend is Veganaise, produced by Follow Your Heart, made with raw and cold pressed grapeseed Oil.

Oils - Buy only cold-pressed varieties. In cold-pressed oils, the seed, nut, grain or vegetable is not heated or bleached to extract the oil. Flaxseed, Macadamia Nut, Coconut, Grapeseed, sesame, and extra virgin olive oil are often cold-pressed. Remember that these are condiments, so use them sparingly and preferably raw. Oils kept at 215 degrees for 15 minutes or longer, (excluding Macadamia, Coconut, Grapeseed, and Avocado oil), have proven to cause arteriosclerosis, or hardening of the arteries.

> ❖ Try sautéing in water or broth instead of oil. If you choose to sauté, cook, grill, stir-fry, or bake with oil -- the healthiest choices include Coconut, Grapeseed, Avocado, or Macadamia Nut oil. There is no danger of those deadly trans-fatty acids and free radicals forming as they can with other cooking oils. Olive oil is best used raw and not heated. Refer to Chapter 8 to learn more about oils.

Seasonings

Herbs and Spices - Avoid irradiated herbs and spices, and try to buy organic. The label should inform you whether they have been irradiated and whether they are certified organic.

Sea Salt – My two favorite types of sea salt are **Himalayan Salt** and **Celtic Sea Salt.** These salts retain their very rich mineral and trace mineral content.

Sea Vegetables - These are powerhouses of nutrition. Collectively they contain 56 known minerals and trace elements essential to our body. They provide high amounts of calcium, iodine, iron, magnesium, and potassium. Sea vegetables also contain another interesting element -- sodium alginate. This mineral takes on a salty jell-like consistency and attaches to heavy metals in our stomach and intestinal tract. It helps eliminate environmental and radioactive contaminants through the bowel. Seaweeds have been proven to reduce these toxins 50-80 percent. They are also healing to the mucus membranes, aid in digestion, help the flexibility and mobility of joints and promote healthy skin.

Dulce - Dulce is a red sea algae with a mild salty flavor. Grind it up for use in sauces, soups, and salads.

Nori - (Nori Sheets) A green algae that is pressed into sheets which can be used as wrappers for rice and vegetables. It can also be crumbled over salads and dishes.

Agar - Agar is a sea plant that has gelatin-like properties and is used to replace gelatin in desserts. It is usually marketed in flakes. To use, mix three tablespoons of Agar into one cup of liquid. Bring the mixture to a boil, stirring constantly. Cook for five minutes, and then completely cool before adding to pieces of raw fruit. It is great for raw fruit pies.

Kuzu Root: Kuzu is a versatile starch that may be used in recipes calling for a thickener such as sauces, gravies, soups, desserts, and beverages. To prepare: For each cup of liquid, use 1 tablespoon kuzu dissolved in 2 tablespoons of cold liquid. Stirring, add dissolved kuzu to your recipe and heat until clear.

Food Shopping List Sample

1.   Sprouted bread - <u>Alvarado</u>, Ezekiel, Trader Joe's brand – found at health food stores
     & Trader Joe's.
2.   Veganaise (non-dairy mayonnaise) – has a purple label & made with raw grapeseed oil, found at health food stores.
3.   Brown rice & other whole grain and sprouted crackers – found at health food stores &
     Trader Joe's.
4.   Almond, Goat, or Hemp milk found at health food stores & Trader Joe's.
5.   Organic whole grains such as quinoa, buckwheat, brown rice, millet, spelt and barley –found at health food stores.
6.   Coconut Aminos and Nama Shoyu – found at most health food stores.
7.   Celtic Sea Salt and Himalayan Salt – found at most health food stores.
8.   Goat yogurt (fruit juice sweetened) – found at health food stores & Trader Joe's.
9.   Fruit juice sweetened yogurt that is organic (look for un-pasteurized)– found at health food stores.

10.   Raw goat cheese by Alta Dena and Wild Wood – found at health food stores.
11.   Pasta: Vita Spelt pasta, Ezekiel Sprouted pasta, Quinoa pasta, & Brown Rice pasta—found at health food stores.
12.   Ezekiel sprouted corn and multi grain tortillas.
13.   Raw nuts/seeds, organic – soak & sprout when possible.
14.   Cream of brown rice, buckwheat, steel cut oats, quinoa and other whole grain hot cereals – found at health food stores.
15.   Organic cold cereals such as Kashi, Nature's Path, Familia, etc. made with spelt, brown rice, quinoa, amaranth, buckwheat, and oats, are healthier choices for cold cereal (make sure they are naturally sweet & no sugar added) – found at Trader Joe's or health food stores.
16.   Lots of organic vegetables and fruits!
17.   Dairy free dressing by "Annies" – found at health food stores and Trader Joe's.
18.   Green Super-food blends (wheat grass, barley grass, alfalfa, kelp, spirulina, chlorophyll, algaes (especially blue-green algae, etc.).
19.   Wild Salmon, Halibut, Sea Bass, Snapper, Mahi Mahi and various other fish (avoid farm-raised).
20.   Wild/Free range and organic poultry, eggs and beef (nitrate/nitrite free).
21.   Red Super-food blends (powdered blends of berries such as Acai, blueberry, Goji, Schizandra, Cranberry, Pomegranate, Mangosteen, Bilberry, etc.).
22.   Sweeteners such as raw honey, organic maple syrup, Yacon Syrup, Xylitol and Stevia can generally be found at health food stores and sometimes Trader Joe's.
23.   Raw/Un-pasteurized & organic fresh juices – Available at Trader Joe's & various natural food markets.
24.   Raw, unrefined, cold-pressed and organic coconut, grapeseed, macadamia nut and olive oil – found at health food stores and occasionally Trader Joe's.
25.   Raw & organic nut butters – found at health food stores.
26.   Tea: Yerba Mate, green tea (Matcha), herbal teas, Rooibos Tea – found at Trader Joe's & health food stores

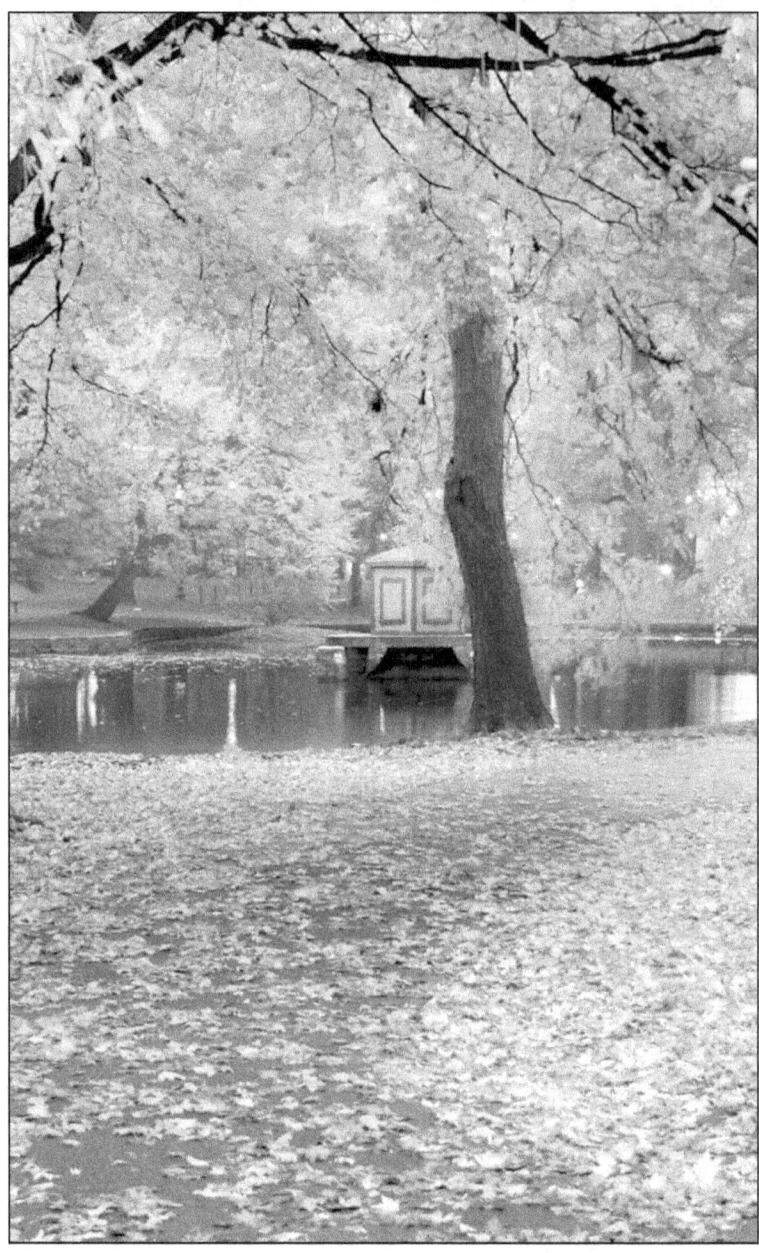

"The time to relax is when you don't have time for it."
~ Attributed to both Jim Goodwin and Sydney Harris

CHAPTER NINETEEN

Natural Alternative Substitutions

Baking Powder:
1 part baking soda with 2 parts cream of tartar and 2 parts arrow-root powder. (Example: 1 tsp. of baking soda, plus 2 tsp. of cream of tartar, plus 2 tsp. of arrowroot powder = 5 tsp. of baking powder.)

Butter:
For sautéing use, coconut oil, grapeseed oil, macadamia nut oil, water with tahini, Nama Shoyu, or Coconut Aminos. For spreads use nut butters, coconut oil or avocado. In baking use equal amounts of applesauce, banana, coconut oil (my favorite), or grapeseed oil.

Buttermilk:
Replace with equal amounts of almond milk with a small amount of nutritional yeast whipped in. You can add a couple splashes lemon juice to get that tang you find in buttermilk

Cheese:
Replace with equal amounts of goat, almond, or raw cow's milk cheese. Goat cheese is much easier to digest than cow's milk. In cooking sauces add nutritional yeast for a cheesy flavor. For cottage or ricotta cheese, try using ground walnuts or tofu mixed with nutritional yeast and lemon juice. For raw foods try a seed/nut yogurt. To replace cream cheese use soy cream cheese and egg-less mayonnaise (Veganaise). Try crumbled and seasoned tempeh or raw goat milk feta on a salad to replace feta cheese crumbles.

Roatsed Cocoa Powder:
Replace with equal amounts of carob powder or raw cacao powder.

Chocolate Sauce:
Try blending cacao powder with coconut oil and Agave. Use about ½ cup cocoa powder to ¼ cup coconut oil and then add Agave syrup to taste.

Coffee:
Try Yerba Mate Tea (naturally has some caffeine but is very cleansing, metabolism stimulant, and appetite suppressant), Calli tea (a *Sunrider* product), Matcha Green Tea, Green Tea, Chicory Root, or other herb teas.

Corn Starch:
Replace with arrowroot powder. Use 1½ times the amount called for. It may thin out if stirred or heated excessively. Stir gently and cook only until thickened. Tapioca Flour is a great replacement in baked goods. In raw desserts, use agar, kuzu or psyllium.

Heavy Cream:
Substitute equal amounts of unsweetened Almond Cream, coconut milk or coconut oil. For sauces, use equal amounts of coconut milk or dissolve 2 tablespoons of tahini in ½ cup water and replace with equal amounts.

Sour Cream:
Replace with equal amounts of plain goat or soy yogurt or try the recipe at my site for the raw Sunflower Dip.

Eggs:
One egg equals 1 tablespoon of soy lecithin dissolved in 1 tablespoon of water, or use packaged egg replacer powder per instructions. For scrambled eggs you can use crumbled sprouted tofu instead. Also, ¼ cup egg whites equal about 1 egg.

Flour:
Coconut flour has become my favorite but works best when combined with tapioca flour. Try using part Tapioca Flour and whole grain flour to make lighter/fluffier baked goods. Use only whole grain flour when using a grain-based flour. To replace 1 cup of flour with oat, rice, quinoa, and other whole grain flours, use 1½ cups. Use same amounts of spelt flour as whole wheat.   Use organic and if possible, soaked, sprouted and dehydrated grains. Grinding your own grains provides the best and most nutritious flours.

Gelatin:
For desserts and sauces use 2 tablespoons of flaked agar to 3½ cups of liquid. If using granulated agar, use half as much.

Fresh Garlic:
1 medium clove of garlic equals 1 teaspoon of minced garlic or ½ teaspoon of granulated garlic powder.

Fresh Herbs:
1 tablespoon of fresh herbs is equal to 1 teaspoon of the dried herb.

Dairy-based Milk:
Use equal amounts of coconut, hemp, or almond milk. For sweeter recipes, try coconut milk or fruit milks such as banana, mango, apple, cantaloupe, watermelon, strawberry, blueberry, grapes, peach or apricot milk (the fruit blended with water or coconut milk.

Black Strap Molasses:
Use equal amounts of barley malt syrup, rice bran syrup or sorghum molasses.

Salt:
For 1 teaspoon of processed salt use 1/3 to ½ teaspoon of Celtic Sea Salt or equal amounts of kelp or dulce. In cooking, try chickpea miso, Nama Shoyu, or Coconut aminos.

Soy Sauce:
Use equal amounts of Nama Shoyu or Tamari or slightly more of Coconut Aminos.

Oil - Baked sweets:
Replace with equal amounts of applesauce, or ground up raw, peeled and cored apples. Use equal amounts of coconut, grapeseed or macadamia nut oil. Also try using equal amounts of fruit juice-sweetened jam or a mashed banana. If two or more cups of oil are required, try using half ground nuts and half fruit.

Oil - Non-sweetened baked goods:
For crusts, breads or rolls use equal amounts of finely ground soaked nuts mixed with 2 teaspoons of water, or equal amounts of Coconut, Grapeseed or Macadamia Nut oil.

Oil - Sauces, gravies and dressings:
For ½ cup of oil use 1/4 cup tahini, Coconut, Grapeseed or Macadamia Nut Oil, finely ground nuts or nut butters blended with 1/8 cup of water.

Sugar - Baking or Raw:
Use equal amounts of maple syrup, yacon syrup or honey, or slightly more of an organic syrup. Use about 1/3 more of Xylitol to sugar (1 cup sugar = 1 1/3 cup Xylitol). Reduce the liquid in the recipe by 1/4 cup per cup of honey or syrup used. Try using equal amounts of date or maple sugar. Use equal amounts of fruit puree.

Sugar - Drinks:
Use 4 to 5 drops of Stevia per 1 cup or maple syrup to taste. Use about 1/3 more of Xylitol to sugar, which dissolves in hot or cold liquids. Honey dissolves easily in hot liquids. For cold liquids, dissolve honey in a small amount of hot water and then add to the cold liquid.

Sugar - Powdered:
Place maple or raw sugar in a grain grinder and grind to a powder.

Canned Tomatoes:
Use fresh tomatoes, chopped or pureed according to the recipe. When cooking tomatoes, add them as your last step—preferably when the heat is turned off. To thicken your recipe, add 2-3 tablespoons of flour at the beginning of your preparation.

Water Chestnuts:
Also try Jerusalem artichokes.

Yogurt:
In cooked foods use equal amounts of soft tofu, plain coconut yogurt or goat yogurt. For raw recipes use equal amounts of seed/nut yogurt.

Meat:
    Sandwiches: For burgers, try one of my recipes at www.justgoodenergy.com. Grilled veggies are a yummy replacement – especially grilled Portobello mushrooms. Thinly sliced and seasoned tempeh is great for sandwiches or wraps. For sandwich spreads try my paté recipes or humus.

Main Dishes: Try substituting with grilled eggplant, sautéed mushrooms, and/or seasoned and grilled tempeh or sprouted tofu.

Tofu or Tempeh: Tofu is sold in moist blocks (choose the sprouted tofu) and tempeh is sold in a more firm block (easily crumbled). Try marinating and broiling with seasonings. Tofu and tempeh can be crumbled, thinly sliced, or cubed and then marinated.

Barbecue and Chicken-flavored beef marinade:
Use beef/chicken flavored vegetarian broth (chemical-free), natural organic barbecue sauce, Worcestershire sauce, onion powder, miso and garlic powder.

Sweet and sour marinade:
Mix pineapple juice with teriyaki sauce and a dash of cayenne.

Other marinades:
Tofu and tempeh are very versatile and easily take on flavors within a half-hour of marinating. Be creative. Try mixing different spices with Liquid Aminos or other flavorful liquids and sauces to create your own marinades. Tofu is sold in moist blocks and tempeh is sold in a more firm block (easily crumbled). Choose the more firm block of tofu, which enables it to absorb the marinade better. With tempeh, simply crumble it up, stir in the marinade and bake in the oven.

Part IV

Soaking & Sprouting

Chapter 20
Soaking & Sprouting Procedures

Chapter 21
Indoor Gardening

CHAPTER
TWENTY

Soaking & Sprouting
Procedures

Any nut, seed, grain, or legume that you are going to soak and/or sprout should be organic, without preservatives or additives and raw and whole. It is best to not over-sprout, as the flavor often becomes bitter. Grain tails should be no longer than the grain itself.

Soaking

To soak most seeds, nuts, grains, or legumes, rinse them thoroughly in a colander or a fine-mesh strainer. Fill a quart jar no more than half full and cover with water, ideally, to about 3 inches above the seeds. Cover the jar loosely with a lid or mesh netting. Allow the seeds and nuts to soak for about 8-12 hours and legumes and grains for about 24 hours (See the soaking/sprouting chart for specifics on nuts, seeds, grains, and legumes.)

After soaking, use a strainer to drain away the soaked water and hulls. Rinse the seeds with fresh filtered water and drain well. Now you are ready to sprout. Those grains, seeds, or nuts that do not naturally sprout should be rinsed thoroughly and refrigerated in covered jars.

Sprouting

After completing the soaking procedure, secure a wire mesh screen or a fine mesh-type cloth over the top of the jar. Wide mouth canning jars with screw bands to hold mesh in place work great for this. Rest the jar at a 30-45 degree angle for about 12-24 hours. (See our soaking/sprouting chart for specifics.)

It is best to cover the jar with a towel or to sprout the seedlings in a dark or dimly lit area to fool them into thinking they are underground! Some sprouts, such as alfalfa, require sunlight the last one or two days of sprouting to receive the all-important chlorophyll from the sun. It is important that the sproutlings are well ventilated; the sprouts should not block the opening of the sprouting jar.

Some people prefer to use sprout bags, baskets or tray-type sprouters. If you choose to use a tray-type sprouter, spread the soaked seeds evenly over the bottom of the tray to assure even growth. Cover the tray with a lid to keep out the sunlight and the sprouts will grow evenly like grass. During sprouting, sproutlings need to be rinsed with filtered water about twice a day. Make sure the sprouts are well drained. They need an even amount of water and air. Don't let them dry out, but too much water left on the sprouts can cause spoilage and mold.

Soaking Dried Fruits

To return dried fruits to their original live form, you only need to soak them. Try to purchase organic un-sulphured dried fruits. Sulfur is a preservative that keeps dried fruit looking beautiful; so whenever a dried fruit looks pretty, beware! Soak all dried fruits in water before eating. If you don't use the soaked fruit right away, refrigerate it in the soaking water in glass jars. Use both the fruit and the soaking water in recipes. Most soaked, dried fruits retain their freshness up to 1½ weeks.

Raisins and Currants
Soak these for 30 minutes to 2 hours, depending on intended use. To quick-soak, use warm water.

Prunes, figs, pears, peaches, apricots, pineapple, and any dried berries
Soak these in filtered water overnight, or for about 8 hours.

CHAPTER
TWENTY-ONE

Your Kitchen Can Be Your Garden

In today's lifestyle, most of us, including me, are dependent on obtaining produce from local grocers and farmers markets. As you become more skilled in the kitchen as it pertains to soaking, sprouting, and juicing, you may decide that you want to explore growing your own grasses for juicing, and your own greens and sprouts for salads. It is actually fairly easy, and can be very enjoyable, just as anything is when you are creating something yourself. It can also be a cost effective alternative to the often inflated prices for organic produce and fresh wheat grass. Below are the steps to creating your own indoor garden. The Sprouting Chart at the end of this chapter gives you exact tips on how long to sprout and the expected yield.

Items to Purchase
- Organic topsoil and peat moss or screened compost.
- 12-16 trays. Hard plastic cafeteria type or plant trays from a nursery are good. Line the trays with paper before pouring in the soil. With cafeteria trays, you don't have to worry about dripping water all over the kitchen floor.
- Wide mouth jars with screw bands or large rubber bands, and nylon mesh or cheesecloth.

Amounts
- Dry seeds: A normal 10 x14 inch tray holds:
- Wheat Berries, rye, barley, oat = 1½ cups
- Sunflower Seeds = 2 - 2 1/4 cups
- Buckwheat = 1-1 1/4 cups

You can split a tray and plant it with one cup sunflower seeds and ½ cup buckwheat groats.

Day 1
- Sort out the broken, chipped or cracked seeds and wash the remainder well in filtered water. Place the seeds in wide-mouth jars and cover them with water, about 3-4 inches above the seeds. Soak for 12 hours.
- Drain the seeds after soaking and rinse well.
- Place the jar at a 45-degree angle for about 12 hours.
- When you see the sprout or tail beginning to appear, they are ready to plant.

Day 2-5
- Mix equal amounts of damp peat moss and topsoil in a barrel or container.
- Spread this mixture about 1 inch deep on the bottom of the tray.
- Work the soil with your hands so that it is loose and smooth.
- Form trenches around the edges of the tray to catch any excess water.
- Spread the sprouted seeds on top of the soil so the seeds touch one another on all sides, but preferably not on top of each other. (Don't worry if they overlap--they will grow anyway.)

❖ All seeds should have access to the soil, forming a thick carpet.
❖ Wet the soil thoroughly, without forming pools of water.
❖ Don't make it muddy.
❖ Cover the tray with another tray or natural cloth.

Keep the seed trays in darkness for about three days or until the sprouts push up the tray cover.

Day 6
❖ Remove the tray covers or cloth.
❖ Water the greens and set them in indirect sunlight.
❖ Before watering the wheat grass, sprinkle it with a tablespoon of powdered or flaked kelp. This adds more trace minerals and iodine.
❖ Continue watering the greens daily.
❖ We recommend watering each morning, or every other day in damp weather.
❖ Keep the soil moist, but do not saturate.
❖ If a tray dries out, do not soak it.
❖ This will shock the young plants. Just moisten the soil and make sure that it does not dry out again.

Day 7
❖ Now the greens are usually at their peak. Buckwheat and sunflower greens will be about 5-7 inches tall and wheat grass about 7-8 inches tall. (Wheatgrass usually takes 6-12 days to mature).
❖ For a sweeter sprout, harvest the sunflower grain before the second set of leaves or shoots appear.
❖ When harvesting, cut as close to the root as possible without pulling out clumps of soil. The base is where the majority of the vitamins are stored.
❖ You may wish to grow a second crop in the same soil. The second crop is never as thick as the first.
❖ Sunflower and buckwheat will not grow a second crop, but those seeds that did not have a chance to grow will now have the opportunity.

Use the wheat grass and greens as soon as possible after harvesting. Some store unused portions of the greens or grass, wrapped in damp paper towels, in plastic bags in the refrigerator.

❖ **Helpful Tips**
A wood dish rack set on a cafeteria tray makes an excellent rack for draining and sprouting your seeds. Don't worry about doing each of these steps perfectly; they will turn out fine anyway.

This is a fun activity for the kids. Get them involved!

Find a routine that works for you. For example, set up seeds to soak overnight, drain and rinse them in the morning, and then plant that evening. If you do not get a chance to plant the seeds that evening, make sure you give them a good rinse and plant them in the morning.

Recommended Daily Amounts

When you start drinking wheat grass, you should take one ounce a day on an empty stomach--first thing in the morning. Drink the wheat grass slowly and swish it around in your mouth so that it mixes with your saliva. Wait at least 30 minutes before eating or drinking other foods. Gradually increase your consumption. Some people drink as much as 4-5 ounces a day. To make it more palatable, during juicing try adding one or two fresh mint leaves per ounce.

Chlorophyll

The chlorophyll in plants resembles red blood cells in our own bodies. It is made up of similar elements, so it is ideal as a food-medicine for the human body. Chlorophyll is produced in plants through the absorption of solar energy, air, water and minerals from the earth.

Chlorophyll cleanses, builds body cells, and is very healing to the human body. It can help reduce blood pressure, reverse anemia, relieve arthritic conditions, help to unclog arteries and helps the wave-like motion in the digestive tract to move the food along. Chlorophyll gives you energy and stamina.

Organically grown grasses are the best sources for this wonderful healing liquid. We recommend 1-3 ounces of wheat grass juice, 1-2 glasses of fresh green vegetable and sprout juices, and at least one large salad consisting of sprouts, greens and a variety of vegetables per day.

Prior to World War II, chlorophyll, in the form of grasses and extracts, was used as an antiseptic and as a poultice. It was given to relieve pain for the treatment of ulcers and many skin diseases. It was reported that in thousands of cases there was an improvement or healing. However, after World War II, antibiotics and chemical antiseptics replaced chlorophyll.

Today, health officials are once again recognizing chlorophyll's wonderful healing capabilities.

One of our friends had lost most of her vision in one eye due to parasites, and her other eye was beginning to be affected. The medical profession was treating her with various antibiotics as well as using chlorine as eyewash. The problem persisted and, aside from being very painful, she feared that she would lose her vision completely. She began using wheat grass juice as an eye wash and changed her diet, including drinking 1-3 ounces of wheat grass juice a day. Within three weeks, more than 70 percent of her vision had returned, and she now sees perfectly.

Used internally or externally, chlorophyll helps us stay healthy!

Sprouting Chart

Seed	Hours to Soak	Sprouting Time (Days)	Length of Tails (Inches)	Times/ Day to Rinse	Notes
Alfalfa	6 - 8	4 - 6	1 - 1 1/2	2	3 Tablespoons of seed fills an entire quart jar. Place in the sunlight for the last 1-2 days, before harvesting
Clover	6 - 8	4 - 6	1 - 1 1/2	2	3 Tablespoons of seed fills an entire quart jar. Place in the sunlight for the last 1-2 days, before harvesting
Garlic, Chive, Onion	6 - 8	4 - 6 (By Itself)	1-1 1/2	2	Best if mixed with alfalfa/clover during soaking, in small amounts. Takes 6-14 days if sprouting by itself
Fenugreek	8	3 - 4	1/2 - 1	2	Pungent flavor, best if mixed with other seeds
Sesame	4-6	1 day (optional)	No tails	2	Slightly sprout, but no tails
Sunflower	4-6	1	0 - 1 1/2	2	Sprout easily, often times with just soaking, will even sprout in the refrigerator If it sprouts too long, becomes bitter
Pumpkin (Papita)	4-6	1 day (No visible sprout)	No tails		Do not sprout at all
Chia Seeds	15 min	1 day	0-1/4		Stir constantly for 5 minutes while soaking
Nut					
Almond	8-10	0	No tails		Swells up and appears sprouted, but is not
Cashews	8-12	0	No tails		Does not sprout. Rinse 2-3 times during soaking
Hazel Nut	8 - 12	0	No tails		Does not sprout
Macadamia	8 - 12	0	No tails		Does not sprout
Pecan	8 - 12	0	No tails		Does not sprout
Pine Nut	4-6	0	No tails		Does not sprout. Soaking helps to break down their acid
Walnut	8 - 12	0	No tails		Does not sprout. Soaking helps to break down their acid

162 -

Legume	Hours to Soak	Sprouting Time (Days)	Length of Tails (Inches	Times/ Day to Rinse	Notes
Adzuki	12 - 15	3	1/2 - 1	2 - 3	Small red bean from China
Black (Turtle) Bean	24	2	1/2 - 1	2 - 3	
Garbanzo (Chick Pea)	12-15	2 - 3	1/2	2 - 3	
Lentil (Brown, Green, Red)	12	2	1/4 - 3/4	2 - 3	Develop slight tails with even just soaking
Mung	12	3 - 5	1/2 - 1 1/2	2 - 3	Commonly known as "Bean Sprouts"
Green Pea	12	2 - 3	1/2	2 - 3	Make sure and use whole peas
Pinto Bean	24	2 - 3	1/2 - 1	2 - 3	Difficult to digest
Soy Bean	15 - 24	2 - 3	1/2 - 1	2 - 3	Most difficult legume to digest

Legume	Hours to Soak	Sprouting Time (Days)	Length of Tails (Inches	Times/ Day to Rinse	Notes
Grain					
Amaranth	6 - 8	2 - 3			
Scotch Barley	24	1 day or less	May not have a tail	2	Use only Scotch Barley and not Pearl Barley (It is unrefined)
Millet	8 - 12	2 - 3	1/4	2 - 3	
Oat Groats	12 - 18	2 - 3 If unsteamed)	1/4	2 - 3	If steamed during process, will not sprout
Brown Rice	24 - 30	1 - 2	1/4	2 - 3	After soaking, place in a colander for sprouting
Rye	18 - 24	2 - 3	1/4 - 1/2	2 - 3	Try mixing with wheat
Spelt	24	2 - 3	1/4 - 1/2	2 - 3	A type of wheat
Wheat	24	2 - 3	1/4 - 1/2	2 - 3	Spring wheat is soft and winter wheat is harder, which is better for sprouting
Quinoa	6-8	2	1/8	2 - 3	Does not sprout very much

Bibliography & Reference Reading

Arlin, Stephen, Fouad Dini and David Wolfe. *Nature's First Law: The Raw-Food Diet*. San Diego, CA: Maul Brothers Publishing, 1996.

Balch, James and Phyllis. *Prescription for Nutritional Healing.* Avory Publishing Group, 2000.

Ballentine, Rudolph, M.D. *Transition to Vegetarianism An Evolutionary Step.* Honesdale, Pennsylvania: The Himalayan International Institute of Yoga Science and Philosophy of the U.S.A, 1987.

Blaylock, Russell L., M.D. *Excitotoxins The Taste that Kills.* Santa Fe, New Mexico: Health Press, 1997.

Bohager, Tom. *Enzymes: What the Experts Know.* Prescott, AZ: One World Press, 2006.

Challem, Jack and Berkson, Burton, M.D. and Smith, Melissa Diane. *Syndrome X.* New York, NY: John Wiley & Sons, Inc., 2000.

Cheraskin, E., M.D., D.M.D. and Ringsdorf, W.M. Jr., D.M.D. and Clark, J.W., D.D.S. *Diet and Disease.* Keats Publishing, Inc., 1995.

Christopher, Dr. John R.., M.H., N.D. *Regenerative Diet.* Provo, Utah: Christopher Publications, 1987.

Christopher, Dr. John R.. *Herbal Home Health Care.* Provo, Utah: Christopher Publications, 1998.

Cichoke, Anthony J. *Enzymes & Enzyme Therapy.* D.C.: Keats Publishing Inc., 1994.

Colbin, AnneMarie. *Food and Healing.* New York, NY: Ballantine Books, 1996.

D'Adamo, Peter J., Dr. *Eat Right 4 Your Type.* New York, NY: G.P. Putnam's Sons, 1996.

Diamond, Marilyn. *The American Vegetarian Cook Book.* New York, N.Y: Warner Books, 1990.

Diamond, Harvey and Marilyn. *Fit for Life II.* New York, N.Y: Warner Books, 1988

Eades, Mary Dan, M.D. *The Doctor's Complete Guide to Vitamins and Minerals.* New York, NY: Dell Publishing, 1994.

Factors of Life, Weight Management, Issue #6010. San Antonio, Texas: Michael's Naturopathic Programs, 1996.

164 -

Factors of Life, Glucose Metabolism Factors, Issue #1200. San Antonio, Texas: Michael's Naturopathic Programs, 1996.

Fadia, Vijay. *Nature's Remedies.* Torrance, CA: Homestead Schools, Inc., 1999.

Haas, Elson M, M.D., *Staying Healthy With Nutrition.* Berkeley, CA: Celestial Arts, 1992.

Hobbs, Christopher. *Foundations of Health, Healing with Herbs & Foods.* Loveland, Colorado: Botanica Press, 1992.

Howell, Dr. Edward. *Food Enzymes for Health & Longevity.* Twin Lakes, Wisconsin: Lotus Press, 1994.

Hoiner-Bey, Herb, N.D. *The Healing Power of Flax.* Topanga, CA: Freedom Press, 2004.

Kirschmann, Gayla and John. *Nutrition Almanac Fourth Edition.* New York, NY: McGraw-Hill, 1996.

Michael Klaper, M.D. *Vegan Nutrition: Pure and Simple.* Paia, Maui, HI: Gentle World, Inc., 1998.

Levin, James and Natalie Cederquist. *Vibrant Living.* San Diego, CA: GLO, Inc., 1993.

Mnidell, Earl. *The Vitamin Bible for the 21ˢᵗ Century.* New York, NY: Warner Books, Inc., 1999.

McDougal, John. A. and Mary A. *The New McDougal Cookbook.* Piscataway, NJ: New Century Publishers, Inc., 1985.

Mercola, Joseph, Dr. *Aspartame - What you don't know can hurt you - Why isn't the FDA protecting your health?* 2005.

Mondoa, Emil I. M.D. and Kitei, Mindy. *Sugars That Heal.* New York, NY: Ballantine Publishing Group, 2001.

Page, Linda Rector, N.D., Ph.D. *Healthy Healing.* Healthy Healing Publications, 1998.

Pfeiffer, Carl C., Ph.D., M.D. *Nutrition and Mental Illness.* Rochester, Vermont: Healing Arts Press, 1987.

Robbins, Anthony *Living Health.* Anthony Robbins Company, *Pg. 34 (c) 1999 ARC*

Seibold, Ronald L. *Cereal Grass, What's in it for you?* M.S.: Pines International, Inc., 2003.

Smith, Ed. *Therapeutic Herb Manual.* Williams, Oregon: Ed Smith, 2004.

Stevens, John Robert. *Our Diet and Our Spiritual Walk.* North Hollywood, CA: The Living Word, 1978.

Szekely, Bordeaux. *The Essene Gospel of Peace.* USA: International Biogenics Society, 1981.

Tenney, Louise, M.H. *Nutritional Guide.* Pleasant Grove, Utah: Woodland Publishing, 1997.

The Non-GMO Report, Volume Five, Issue Two. Fairfield, IA: Writing Solutions, Inc., February 2005.

Tierra, Michael, L.Ac., O.M.D. *The Way of Herbs.* New York, NY: Pocket Books, 1998.

Lisa Turner. *Meals That Heal.* Rochester, Vermont: Healing Arts Press, 1996.

Vegetarian Voice, Vol. 19, no. 4. Dolgeville, NY: North American Vegetarian Society, 1993.

Vegetarian Voice, Vol. 21, no. 4. Dolgeville, NY: North American Vegetarian Society, 1993.

Wigmore, Ann. *The Hippocrates Diet and Health Program.* Wayne, NJ: Avery Publishing Group Inc., 1984.

Wigmore, Ann. *The Wheatgrass Book.* Wayne, NJ: Avery Publishing Group Inc., 1985.

Wigmore, Ann. *Recipes for Longer Life.* Wayne, NJ: Avery Publishing Group Inc., 1978.

Referred Websites:

www.AmazingGrass.com
www.holisticmed.com
www.celticseasalt.com/PDF/saltbrochure.pdf
www.uk.geocities.com/veggiemania_org/welcome.htm
www.coconutrtesearchcenter.org/
www.drweil.com
www.enzymedica.com
www.healthfromthesun.com
www.harmonikireland.com
www.lauric.org/functional.html
www.macnutoil.com
www.Naturezone.net
www.rahoorkhuit.net/health/alkaline_vs_acid
www.tonyrobbins.com
www.greenfacts.org/mercury/
www.futurevisions.org/cnn_diet.htm
www.snyderhealth.com/energize.htm
www.mkprojects.com/tl_VibAssess.htm
www.manitobaharvest.com/faq/
www.holisticmed.com
www.mercola.com
www.thecampaign.org
www.darinsnaturals.com
http://air-to-water-blog.com/
www.drmercola.com

www.ingramcontent.com/pod-product-compliance
Lightning Source LLC
Chambersburg PA
CBHW081351280526

45788CB00009B/2838

* 9 7 8 1 4 5 3 7 0 0 8 8 4 *